Dramatherapy with Elders and People with Dementia

Dramatherapy with Elders and People with Dementia illuminates how targeted sessions of dramatherapy can improve the quality of life of elderly people with dementia.

The book takes the reader through the dramatherapy experience of a group of people who display a "feeling intelligence"; a quality that softens distress at vanishing words and clouded memories. Unique in its approach, not only to dramatherapy with elders and people with dementia, but it also presents an essential validation of older people's life stage development.

Rather than being different or "other", Jaaniste paints word pictures to show human qualities such people have in common with their dementia-free contemporaries. Readers will glean insights into the arts therapies, especially creative drama, meeting examples of elder wisdom, wit and resilience in dealing with life, but especially grief, loss and deep questions that come with ageing.

Enriched with vignettes and anecdotes based on rigorous research and measurement, the book will be suitable for adaptation by arts therapists and other allied health professionals who are interested in using person-centred, strengths-based approaches.

Joanna Jaaniste, PhD, has 30 years' experience as a dramatherapist. She has co-created a graduate diploma in dramatherapy and has taught extensively on the MA Art Therapy course at Western Sydney University, Australia.

'This fascinating, innovative contribution to knowledge is invaluable to all those involved in the wellbeing of elders and people with dementia. It provides vivid accounts of research into practice and will inspire and support those working with client experiences of loss, grief or trauma and with the joys of living in the moment and of spirituality.

I am deeply moved by the many examples that illuminate how drama and creativity can be brought into the lives of individuals and groups in ways that enhance their quality of life. The rigour of thinking offered by Jaaniste in her planning and devising, alongside the verve and deep empathy she brings to understanding the impact of her work is inspirational. Chapters on approaches in research, assessment and evaluation will speak to practitioners and researchers in a variety of professions. *Dramatherapy with Elders and People with Dementia* enables learning to happen in a vivid way: reading this text takes us directly into the spaces and activities where change is happening and into the mind of a dramatherapist alive and alert to the meanings of her practice and how her own learning and insight can be shared with us to enable our own discoveries as readers. This is an important, key text in the fields of practice with elders and people with dementia, the arts therapies and dramatherapy. It deserves to be essential reading on professional courses and for practitioners and carers.'

Phil Jones, *Professor, Head of Research Ethics and Governance, UCL Institute of Education (*The arts therapies: A revolution in Healthcare *(2nd ed.) and* Drama as therapy volume 2: Clinical work and research into practice)

'This book summarises art therapies and dramatherapy and how to use such approaches with people living with dementia. This is a valuable textbook for health professionals looking for an alternative psychosocial approach to add to their dementia care toolkit. The chapter exploring intelligence of feeling and dramatherapy is significant in helping readers employ this approach.'

Wendy Moyle, *Professor, Program Director Menzies Health Institute Queensland, Griffith University*

'This book explores Western concepts of aging, dementia and dramatherapy, situated in the Australian context. It speaks to the value of working actively through dramatherapy to create connection with self and other, past and present, to meet the developmental tasks of living and ageing with dementia.'

Kirsten Meyer, *PhD, dramatherapist*

'This book earns Joanna the absolute right to be considered a leading expert in the field of providing effective services with people with dementia. She skilfully combines research, examples of clinical practice and an overview of the ageing processes in this engaging and extremely readable book.'

Madeline Andersen-Warren, *dramatherapist (retired), author and researcher*

Dramatherapy: Approaches, relationships, critical ideas
Series Editor: Professor Anna Seymour

This series brings together leading practitioners and researchers in the field of dramatherapy to explore the practices, thinking and evidence base for dramatherapy.

Each volume focuses on a particular aspect of dramatherapy practice, its application with a specific client group, an exploration of a particular methodology or approach or the relationship between dramatherapy and related field(s) of practice, all informed by ongoing critical analysis of existing and emergent theoretical ideas.

In each case the aim is to develop the knowledge base of dramatherapy as a unique discipline, whilst contextualising and acknowledging its relationship with other arts and therapeutic practices.

As such the series will produce different kinds of books to encompass a spectrum of readers from trainee dramatherapists and arts practitioners to academic researchers engaged in multidisciplinary enquiry.

The field of dramatherapy is expanding internationally and this series aims to respond to emergent clinical and critical needs within practice based and academic settings. These settings are increasingly diverse serving complex needs and demand dynamic and incisive literature to support clinical intervention and as resources for critique.

In this series:

Dramatherapy and Autism
Edited by Deborah Haythorne and Anna Seymour

Dramatherapy and Borderline Personality Disorder
Edited by Nicky Morris

Dramatherapy with Elders and People with Dementia
By Joanna Jaaniste

https://www.routledge.com/Dramatherapy/book-series/DRAMA

Dramatherapy with Elders and People with Dementia

Enabling Developmental Wellbeing

Joanna Jaaniste

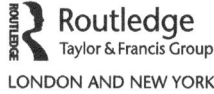
Routledge
Taylor & Francis Group

LONDON AND NEW YORK

Cover image: Shutterstock

First published 2023
by Routledge
4 Park Square, Milton Park, Abingdon, Oxon OX14 4RN

and by Routledge
605 Third Avenue, New York, NY 10158

Routledge is an imprint of the Taylor & Francis Group, an informa business

British Library Cataloguing-in-Publication Data
A catalogue record for this book is available from the British Library

ISBN: 978-1-032-03032-6 (hbk)
ISBN: 978-1-032-03030-2 (pbk)
ISBN: 978-1-003-18632-8 (ebk)

DOI: 10.4324/9781003186328

Typeset in Times New Roman
by KnowledgeWorks Global Ltd.

Contents

11 Conclusion 143

Biography

Dr Joanna Jaaniste

BA(Hons), DipEd, DipDramatherapy, PhD, AThR

Joanna is a registered dramatherapist and Adjunct Fellow at Western Sydney University, where she has researched and lectured on the Master of Art Therapy course over many years. She is the Director of The Dramatherapy Centre, Sydney, which teaches introductory and advanced dramatherapy courses. She has been a founding board member for Australasia of the World Alliance of Dramatherapy for the past six years and has now retired from that position. She has extensive experience in the area of mental health and specialises in dementia. Joanna has a small private practice and is a qualified supervisor. She has lectured and presented in Europe, the USA, South Africa and New Zealand and has published widely on dramatherapy.

Foreword

This very engaging book is full of ideas and information for both general and professional readers. Along with therapists in various modalities, readers with family members who have dementia would find it helpful and interesting, as would many with a recent diagnosis of dementia.

The book has two major, interlinked themes. These are the importance of the model of care and the place of the arts therapies in the lives of people with dementia. Can a quality of life (QoL) model inform practice or whether practice is more dominated by safety concerns outweighing and sometimes replacing QoL considerations? This includes QoL in terms of the individual and not just in terms of an observer or caregiver.

The other major theme is the role the arts therapies can play in enhancing QoL through activities such as singing in choirs, movement with or without music, art which engages the body and mind in creative ways and dramatherapy. The book gives examples from a series of group sessions of dramatherapy, where purposeful engagement with a skilled dramatherapist allowed a sense of community and trust to develop. This process provided the opportunity for the participants to express empathy for themselves and others, and to share key moments of their lives in ways they generally had little opportunity to do.

There are around 50 million people in the world with dementia, and the numbers are increasing. There is no known cure and increasing numbers of people with dementia live in residential/institutional care. The main focus of this care seems to be moving from a QoL perspective to prioritising safety, as indicated in a recent Australian review of aged care facilities. Both are important, but the QoL aspects can be lost when safety becomes the primary concern, with the safety of the body often the focus of all care decisions and a mind-body split reinforced or reintroduced to care design and implementation.

This book makes a strong case for placing QoL as the main criterion around which care is designed and implemented. This includes access to mind-body therapies, supported as they are by neuroscience and arts therapies research. As an experienced dramatherapist, Joanna builds her case around nearly 30 years of experience, her own doctoral research with a group of people with dementia, and the embodied practice of dramatherapy. She is creative in finding an appropriate combination of qualitative and quantitative research approaches to assess this project and to involve group members and their supporters in the evaluation. She makes a compelling case for access to dramatherapy for people with a diagnosis of dementia. The people she worked with for her doctoral research demonstrated that, in dramatherapy groups, people with dementia can access memories, emotions and spiritual connections which are not recognised or encouraged in everyday care, especially in residential care. Those diagnosed with dementia are often separated from the company, the concerns and the support available to many in their age group. This separates them from sharing their common humanity. Dramatherapy focuses on those things we share as people and provides the means to share them, often in funny, creative and stimulating ways.

Dementia is a set of neurological disorders which are often treated as psychiatric conditions. This approach may mask co-existing psychiatric disorders like depression, anxiety and post-traumatic stress disorder, which then may not be separately treated. Such an approach may not consider head injuries from sport or fights or other trauma, or deficits caused by poverty, poor diet and poor general health. There are four main types of dementia, with the most prevalent being Alzheimer's disease (AD), with AD sometimes being an interchangeable term with dementia. Dementia may be present in mild, moderate and severe degrees. The diagnosis of dementia is based on narrowly focused and generally inappropriate cognitive tasks and some of the tasks of daily living, including changes in relationships. Where does that leave other functions and needs, such as to be part of a family, to be part of a group with similar interests, to love and be loved and respected, to have a place in the world, to have emotional and spiritual needs recognised? What about Indigenous people? Are they lost in translation? The care available seldom offers the opportunity for these needs to be recognised and for the individual to have recognition and respect for the way they have lived and loved during their lives. There are potential language and cultural barriers in diagnostic practice and alternative explanations for changes in social participation due to deafness and deteriorating eyesight. There may not be recognition of the existence of an inner life or the value of memories from the more distant past. A life story could add more meaning to diagnosis. The emphasis is often on loss and deficit, which reinforces the need for a QoL approach which might be used to provide potentially life-affirming activities.

How robots or virtual pets or other types of artificial intelligence may be used in care settings will depend on the model. Will they be used as minders, diverting staff to more managerial or paper tasks, thus reducing human contact; or will they be used for routine tasks to deliberately free staff to have more human and stimulating interaction with elderly residents?

While there is some early onset dementia, it is generally a disorder of older age, and initially may be hidden within other sensory, neurological and physical deterioration associated with the older life stages.

Within a life stage model, from between 60 and 70 years of age, adults enter an early phase of older adulthood, between about 70 and 80, they are in the middle stage of older adulthood and from the later 80s onward they are in the older adult stage. Through these stages, people experience many changes, several of which are associated with loss. Loss of loved partners and friends, loss of loved ways of life, of work, of connection; loss of physical strength and ability and often decline in health and greater need of medical, social and family support. Ideally, older adults find they now have time, previously filled with work and responsibility, to engage in new aspects of life and previously unexplored aspects of themselves. With death as an unscheduled end stage, its inevitability may become more of a companion leading to a new appreciation of one's life, a greater acknowledgement of the roles that each person has played, a reconciliation with mistakes made and a celebration of achievements gained. All of this occurs in the context of relationships – at home, at work, within the family and with oneself at other life stages. This often allows for response and contemplation as one scans or reviews one's life, often with shared memories and laughter, tears and love. This might be seen as the older years offering opportunity to embrace a fuller humanity. To claim the recognition of a life fully if not richly led, to have and express regret, but to attain a balance of satisfaction at having lived a full range of human experience can be fulfilling indeed.

Those diagnosed with dementia are often excluded from the opportunity to remember and be remembered in a loving review of their life by not being able to recall, not being expected to access the memory and by being increasingly removed from the kind of stimulation, and company of their peers, which allows some of this to occur.

In this important book, Joanna starts from the viewpoint that this is a group of people who have the same life stage needs as their peers, from whom they are separated by their diagnosis and what this means, and by the segregation which largely occurs following diagnosis. They are separated by what they cannot do or how they cannot participate, rather than included by the things they share and can do.

What can dramatherapy offer in this situation? First, there is membership of a group, albeit a time limited one. There is the acceptance, by the dramatherapist and a range of supporters, of possible limitations or difficulties and offering specific actions to recognise these, giving individual support in a way that enables group members to participate fully in the group activities. In these circumstances, Joanna found participants were able to self-advocate and show that they could have a voice in the world.

They demonstrated knowledge and awareness of their own essential personality and, from that, could relate to and support other group members. They showed a clear ability to express ideas and feelings through the dramatherapy and demonstrated resilience in the light of unhappy or traumatic memories.

These experiences occurred through structures and actions that most dramatherapists consider routine, but they are routine because they are sequenced, and they are supported by neuroscience. Sequenced routines help people to join as a group and to achieve outcomes together. It enables them to relax with each other and with themselves in games and warm-ups; to begin to find a physical voice and then to give voice to what matters to them; to have fun and to express their emotions.

These group participants played roles in stories they were presented with, then in their own stories. They were playful with roles and personalities, creating personas to carry the stories forward within a dramatherapy framework, which allows freedom within containment and permits apparent chaos to form a new order within the confines of the dramatherapy space. They found commonalities in experiences and reactions within group, which provided an opportunity to review their lives with acceptance and forgiveness for themselves. At varying levels of engagement, they demonstrated their ability to become involved in the stories of others in the group. They could empathise with these stories and engage with and support other group members and offer support and reassurance. They demonstrated empathy towards themselves, expressed their feelings, and were able to communicate their own remembered emotional experiences. They discovered the positive power of working in a group in supporting others and each others' stories, in bringing stories alive and finding common ground. Reminiscences by group members prompted the memories of other group members. They shared stories, jokes and songs. The stimulation of strong feeling often aided memory. Dementia exists and causes deterioration in brain structure and function, but we could also remember that brain plasticity is real and the right stimulation might illuminate some compensatory skills. The ability to work with others in this group indicates a richer inner life than might be imagined as a person sits still, silent and alone in the dementia facility.

The members of the group and their supporters experienced the positive power of the group in bringing their stories alive. The supporters saw an intelligence of feeling in action in the group members' interpersonal connections. The participants worked together with the essential humanity of this life stage with generosity and kindness.

The stories and the research outlined in this book make a strong case for opportunities to be provided for people with dementia to engage with dramatherapy, as a contained and secure way to face life problems, resolve internal conflicts and express strong emotions. They underline the importance of a person-centred approach which honours a long life, lived as well as possible and with family and carers providing QoL, with stimulating experiences and relationships still possible.

Caroline Miller
PG Dip. Dramatherapy; B.Phil; MA,
PG Dipl. Clinical Psychology
Editor: *Assessment and outcomes in the arts therapies: A person-centred approach.*
Arts therapists in multidisciplinary settings: Working together for better outcomes.
Arts therapies in international settings: Informed by neuroscience and research (with Mariana Torkington).

Preface

This book has been a privilege to write, and I owe its existence to the generosity of the people who had lived experience of dementia at various stages and gave so much of their goodwill to the project on which much of the book is based. As a dramatherapist who is passionate about her work, I felt beckoned on by this community of elders, to write from a more human perspective than I had done in the past about these courageous human beings and their participation in dramatherapy sessions. I felt it was their right to be firmly included in a developmental view of us as a human species – a topic not emphasised in my doctoral study.

Another reason for writing from a developmental point of view is the fact that I am well past three score years and 10 myself. Later on, in the book, I describe a woman I have been visiting in an aged care home who was not much older than myself and she mirrored my own life stage.

> She sits, bent double in her chair
> Her head upon her tray
> She's not aware that I am there
> I don't know what to say.
> But then I speak and touch her arm
> I'm in the same life stage.
> My own lost words serve to disarm
> Myself – I'm near her age.
> She straightens up and sits erect
> Greeting me with a smile
> I lose my fear, its cold effect
> That froze me for a while.
> The sparkle in those tired eyes
> The willingness to share
> Bring with them our engaging rise
> Creating – being there.

Additionally, and connected with the autoethnographic position I have taken in writing the book, my purpose is to bear witness to my own developmental stage on my life journey. I am a white Anglo-Australian woman who had an English mother and an Australian father, and who grew up in the UK, arriving in Australia in time for my 20th birthday. I am the eldest child of a mother who had dementia, as well as the goddaughter of her sister who also had the disease, both of whom have now crossed the threshold. My godmother died only in 2020 at the age of 104 and had been relatively free of dementia until her late 90s. I celebrate their courage and lived experience, as well as those of my participants in my fieldwork and often wonder whether or not the writing of the book has prepared me for an unknown future of dementia. I find myself filled with gratitude that so far, all that has changed are the physical aches and pains that normally announce the onset of ageing, and rejoice in my good health otherwise.

It has also been important for me to acknowledge my socio-cultural bias as an immigrant in a land whose colonial heritage is ever-present and the expression *post-colonial* has an uncomfortable ring to it when so many of our Indigenous First Peoples are still dispossessed. Incidentally, I have used the term "elder" in the book, a term which I understand to be regarded by gerontologists as stigmatising the older person. Personally, I believe that rejecting this term somehow stigmatises First Peoples. I am grateful to them and their cultures for lending it to us, as it implies a certain wisdom that is present in older people, whether they have dementia or not.

Associated with the dispossession of our First Peoples and the gap between rich and poor that is widening in all first world capitalist countries is the question of privilege and the quality of people's lives, especially as they age. It is a tragedy that the excellent work on person-centred care done in the UK more than 20 years ago has often been given lip service only, despite some shining examples of ethical and consistent initiatives to engage with its values. This is a pity, as person-centred care aligns smoothly with quality of life (QoL) principles. It is a tragedy that our own Aged Care Royal Commission report has not paid attention to this phrase but instead has chosen "quality of safety" as its assessment mantra. This recalls for me the story of a family friend whose elderly parent was being restrained in a wheelchair at his nursing home in case he fell. He asked his children to beg the management to leave him free, as he would rather take the risk of falling out of the chair than be imprisoned in it. This, surely, is the difference between the QoL and the quality of safety. People like him should not have their lives overshadowed by the spectre of management's fear of legal repercussions and instead have adequate care staff in place to protect those they serve. It has been important to address the narrative of possible trauma in earlier life and the danger of re-traumatisation using restraint, which I have done in Chapter 7.

Connected with QoL is the concept of wholism, which I take to mean applying high-quality care and interventions in the areas of body, mind and spirit. In offering dramatherapy, we hope to support participants in moving their bodies in a healthy way, taking on body shapes and stances to express feelings, experiences and various roles. Embodiment as aesthetic expression can be a healthy means to get in touch with self and with feelings rarely expressed. Participants in dramatherapy can also find that their minds open up to past memories, to the here-and-now, and imaginations of the future. This approach can be helpful in reminiscence, knowing what day it is and looking forward to events or visits. Spiritually, dramatherapy lends itself to the perception that we are all spiritual beings and addresses the needs of participants in this regard.

As a transpersonal dramatherapist, I draw inspiration from the work of psychotherapists and thinkers who believe there is more to life and the universe than we can see with our eyes and refer to them in the pages of this book. Like them, I value the vital core of every human being. This core can be understood as a light inside each one, which cannot be extinguished either by illness, misfortune or losing one's way in life. In other words, it cannot be damaged by others or by experience. It is a concept that can be closely aligned with person-centred care, and when we recognise that light in another, it is confirmation that we are here for each other and not just for ourselves. I have defined my understanding of spirituality in Chapter 3 as a pure and true way of being engendered from the recognition of elements or being(s) greater than ourselves. In the service of these mysteries, the self has the ability to connect with others and nature and the faith of participants needs to be honoured and respected. Many people who are now between the ages of 70 and 100 have faith in organised religion, and as therapists it is important to be aware of any biases we hold and be prepared to offer them client-centred approaches to expression of their beliefs.

Finally, I trust you will gain something new from this book, whether you are a dramatherapist or have an alternative specialisation, know a loved one with dementia or are an interested elder. I wish you engaging reading!

Acknowledgements

This book is dedicated to the generous people with dementia who originally volunteered to take part in the dramatherapy fieldwork for my doctoral research, which is the foundation upon which the book has taken shape. They kindly gave permission to include my telling of their stories. I have also benefited from the guidance and assistance of dramatherapist Caroline Miller, who has written a gracious foreword to the book. Her help as an experienced editor and colleague has been of inestimable support. I would also like to thank my friend and colleague Kirsten Meyer, also a dramatherapist, for reading the book in its final stages and offering valuable advice. Thanks also go to my excellent copyeditor, Rachel Le Rossignol, who, true to her name, was the nightingale who achieved greater harmony in writing, not only reviewing every word but often by providing two or three alternatives where needed. A big thank you to Dr Sue Jennings for writing the Afterword and for her developmental Embodiment, Projection and Role paradigm, which has been a gift that has guided me in the application of dramatherapy techniques for this age group.

Special thanks go to Maxine Radus and Dannielle Jackson who have contributed valuable vignettes of their work with older people with dementia. Appreciation also goes to Mauricio LaMadrid for his work with my images and files. Conversations with James Greaves, who assists a man with moderate dementia to connect with others on his computer, have been crucial in helping me understand what a slow and difficult process this can be for someone for whom this is the only way to reach out. I am grateful to Professor Anna Seymour's invitation to write this book in her series, and for her support during the process, as well as Joanne Forshaw, Grace McDonnell and Kalie Koscielak at Routledge for answering my frequent questions. Thanks are extended to my friends and family members for their encouragement, and especially to my husband Rein for his constant support that has helped sustain my passion for this work.

This book was written on the lands of the Gadigal people of the Eora nation, where I live. I acknowledge and pay my respects to elders past, present and emerging.

Chapter 1

Life stages and transitions

This book as a whole, and the present chapter, in particular, aim to show how dramatherapy with people with dementia can be considered from the point of view of life stage development. In 2015, I was asked to write for a collection of chapters presenting the work of dramatherapists from around the world (Jaaniste, 2016). Since I had been interested in life stage development before I ever studied dramatherapy, it seemed apt to combine this concern with a decade of experience offering dramatherapy to people with dementia (Jaaniste, 2013). As dramatherapists, we work like all psychotherapists in the area of being human; in the field of "I and Thou" as Buber defines an authentic relationship (1965, p. 60). When we work with the whole person in body, mind and spirit, we have already said a wholehearted "yes" to the humanity of our clients and their life experience. Their life journeys are influenced by their unique nature as humans with milestones in their development. As a gardener, when we observe a full-blown rose on the briar as an end point, it helps to remember it was once a tightly formed bud and will later be a rosehip. It is also the case with human beings. As for all art therapists, the dramatherapist's own development as well as their understanding of developmental matters are important.

The psychoanalyst Freud had little time for the later life stages and, in fact, eschewed the possibility of fruitful education for the over-50s (1905). Jung, however, saw in his ageing clients the possibility of discovery of meaning and purpose in their later years (Prétat, 1994). An unfortunate overtone in his description of old age was to position it as a second childhood; there were, however, valuable aspects in Jung's work that were missing from that of his predecessors (Jung, 1991). He believed that elderly people could move towards acceptance of wholeness through embracing new aspects of their world. There is a turning inward, he says, in the sense that the elderly can give themselves a chance to consider their life destiny introspectively as it draws towards its close.

Elders could take the opportunity, for instance, of recognising aspects of their animus and anima, the former being a male image in the female psyche and the anima a female image in the male psyche. This could be

DOI: 10.4324/9781003186328-1

achieved with the use of roleplay for people with mild dementia and with projective techniques such as choosing figurines or dress-ups for people whose dementia was at the moderate stage. Male and female characteristics could be shared on cards in a group situation and worked with using either of these techniques. Alternatively, painting could be another way of depicting this separation, as in Gordon-Flower's archetypal work with people with physical disabilities (2020, p. 45). These archetypes represent the "true self" rather than the image we present to others and serve as the primary source of communication with the collective unconscious (Jung, 1991).

Erikson made a considerable and well-known contribution to the debate about the life stages, using a polarised approach for each of his eight levels from birth to later life, defining the final stage of life as "ego integrity versus despair" (1963, p. 268). If the older person could not look back on their life as one of integrity, they were more likely to experience fear of death. Erikson's models imply, for the most part, that autonomy and self-responsibility are the highest stage of development (Malone et al., 2016). Our western societies place a high value on activity leading to productivity, effectiveness and self-sufficiency and there is a danger here. We encumber the elderly with our "value-dependent theories" (Tornstam, 2005, p. 23), especially in the area of research. The fact is that far from being totally independent, all of us, with very few exceptions, are deeply intertwined with, and dependent upon, others. This is especially true of ageing people, whether or not they have dementia.

This question of the significant and interdependent relationship with older people is one that we can all benefit from. The wisdom of experience in the elderly is often acknowledged but not always respected. They have a generous capacity to relate to the very young, and this is usually reciprocated. In Australia and the United Kingdom research has shown that social encounters between the elderly and the very young in day care can increase confidence and encourage bonding (Skropeta et al., 2014; Teater, 2016). Due to our global separation of families over the past 50 years, many families lack grandparents in their neighbourhood, their state, or even in the same country. When these two age groups – children and older people – are brought together, magic can happen.

Older people have long memories where the environment is concerned. They feel more connected than others with patches of forest or bush which are in danger of being cut down or lakes and dams at risk of pollution and want the aesthetic beauty of nature present in their younger years to remain with us. Many maintain gardens until they can physically no longer do so and experience joy in planting, grafting and caring for the natural world.

The elderly are no longer very interested in status and ambition and know how to connect with others on an essentially human level. They remember how, in the past, there were other ways than the more current ones of dealing with a problem, and this gives them greater perspective than the younger person with the furrowed brow, trying to engage with complexity. Shakespeare tells us how the ageing King Lear told his daughter the two of them could while away the time in a relaxed way:

> ... So we'll live,
> And pray, and sing, and tell old tales, and laugh
> At gilded butterflies, ...
> And take upon us the mystery of things,
> As if we were God's spies ...
>   (Shakespeare, 1876, pp. 5.3.11–17)

Erikson's later work on generativity and social involvement in old age softened his views somewhat when he collaborated with his younger wife, Joan M. Erikson, and a much younger clinical and research psychologist, Helen Q. Kivnick (Erikson et al., 1989). Their research revealed a much more resourceful and longer-lasting period of generativity than in Erikson's earlier work.

Joan Erikson considered that a ninth stage was necessary in the scheme of life stages. She wrote the final few paragraphs of *The Life Cycle Completed* (1997) because she realised that the eighth stage had been written long before either of them had reached it. She considered that some traditional cultures had got the balance right, where the elderly were appreciated for their wisdom and their ability to look back to the past and connect with it, as well as having a singular empathic relationship with younger generations. She also promoted Tornstam's (1993) contemplative "gerotranscendence" stage, encapsulating the changes apparent in extreme old age as follows:

1 A feeling of "cosmic communion" with the universe (or spiritual connectedness)
2 Time being circumscribed (the future is limited)
3 Reduced mobility, implying a narrowing of personal space
4 Death being seen philosophically as "the way of all living things"
5 A sense of self expanding to include "a wider range of interrelated others" (Erikson, 1997, p. 124)

The sense of connectedness with the universe pre-supposes a less materialistic, more mature viewpoint. A more relational emphasis might decrease the boundaries between the self and the other. Self-importance might be exchanged for a recognition that we all die, just as plants and animals do. Dramatherapy can help connect with a potential change of attitude by introducing stories where a death takes place, giving participants roles and having time to de-role and reflect on their experience in the drama, as in Chapter 8.

Of course, there are many reasons why people can become burdened by old age during the earlier unfolding of the stages of life. Every decade our society demands more and "better" qualifications for jobs and even unpaid positions in the community such as volunteering. Mental health is declining and there is very often a competitive race to have more or to be more than we are or can be. Climate change is a source of anxiety. These situations can bring suffering – a sense of not feeling good enough, not having enough, or of being one of life's victims. The person may lose the sense of who they are entirely. If, however, during the earlier stages of life, a person has worked towards finding meaning in life's ups and downs, this is less likely to happen. Through study, introspection, the examples of others or with spiritual and psychological help, there can be a freedom from guilt and an exoneration from humiliation which assists them to surmount their problems. I would argue that spirituality, in whatever form it comes to the person, can help lighten their load. A possible life stage approach to therapy would include work on personal values and beliefs at all ages, and with the elderly, another sort of timeline where they contemplate their own changing views at various stages. It would be fascinating to see how a particular issue or challenge manifested in a different form with each life stage.

Spirituality, in its many dimensions is an ever-present wellspring for human beings to draw upon and is available to all. Meaningful activities which involve nature, relationship, the arts, prayer and meditation represent wells which never run dry. Those who have found their values in these activities are more likely to find solace in old age. They may recognise the value of acceptance of a certain amount of suffering and will learn to "suffer with" others and to find meaning in it, which can lead to joy.

Even when this has not been entirely the case in earlier life, the opportunities offered by dramatherapy help to build resilience in the here-and-now. This is especially important for people with dementia, as generally speaking, sad and traumatic experiences come to mind more often than happy ones. More will be said in Chapter 4 about the significance of resilience-building using dramatherapy for them. Dramatherapy can lead people back to a memory of a time when healing of unfairness took place or when a relationship led to curative meaning. This memory may arise from a story about something else entirely in the dramatherapy repertoire and, in turn, become a source of wisdom and acceptance – strong values of the later life stages. I am reminded constantly of such moments by people who have been marginalised, abused or abusers – even those who have been responsible for the death of others. Positively characterised life stages can also be borne in mind when the person has dementia, rather than labels such as "end-stage dementia" (Morrison & Siu, 2000, p. 47) or deterioration (Dementia Australia, 2021) which, although useful, are dominated by the negative symptoms of dementia's various forms. Instead, more positive labels could identify the fact that well-entrenched memories laid down during childhood are the last memories to be lost in dementia. This situation occurs because children's memories are not subject to the short-term or middle-term memory loss characteristic of the process of cognitive disintegration associated with the disease (Weisberg & Wilder, 2001).

Undoubtedly there will be a mixture of positive and negative memories. However, it is not kind or helpful for the therapist to gloss over the difficult ones. There may be pressure from the day centre or facility not to deal with these, as there is a risk of the person needing extra psychological care in a time-poor staff environment. It is important that there is a realisation by managers that a dramatherapist is not a diversional therapist. Meeting with and sharing information with the occupational therapist, nurse or care staff can help to put these memories into context and put after-care in place.

Certain positive aspects of dementia could be, firstly, a sense of humour. For example, a client who was approaching severe dementia asked his doctor, who had some bad news for him, if the doctor himself had dementia. Another aspect is letting go of control, even when the person has been an initiator for most of their life. Interdependence can come as a great gift to the family of such a person. In common with elderly people who do not have dementia, they find contentment in more simple events than in previous life stages. They do not have to fill every silence with chat. They are content to have dinner in a restaurant with a friend or family member without talking the entire time – a fact that is often lost on their younger companion. Another positive sign is forgiveness. In a group of six clients at a retirement village, I noticed that an Anglo-Celtic person who had lost her husband in World War II was at first unwilling to communicate with a German participant. After meeting once a week for eight weeks, she had forgiven this woman for being German and called her "beautiful". At a core familial level, there is a realisation for those who resented their parents for their difficult upbringing that those parents were doing the best they could. For example, Neil's forgiveness of his dead father is referred to later in this book, in Chapter 8. Then there is the unexpected moment of wisdom and clarity, when someone who seems quite forgetful much of the time comes out with a saying or quotation which completely fits the moment or the person to whom it is addressed.

People with dementia may be cognitively impaired, but they possess psychic resources which give them a way of seeing the funny or quirky side of a situation. Their lack of expectations of young children allows them to have fun with them and enjoy a shared love of play. In 2017, the Australian Broadcasting Commission (ABC) made a miniseries where a group of scientists and gerontologists brought 10 elderly people from a care home into a room with 10 preschoolers. They wanted to determine whether connection between the two age groups would bring about positive changes in the elderly people's lives. At the end of six weeks of playing and laughing together, the scientists and gerontologists came to the conclusion their quality of life (QoL) had improved (ABC, 2017). Childlike playfulness is a quality most adults could learn from them, as we do not play often enough. The word "disinhibited" in the medical literature is a pejorative one; applied to the elderly with dementia, however, their willingness to have fun and play can dispel so many of the ills, real or imagined, of growing old. It is this quality which, over all others, attracts them to dramatherapy.

Arts therapies, creativity in life and psychotherapy in the later stages of development

Lievegoed (1997) describes the last phases of life for healthy elders more positively than Erikson, noting that those involved in creativity can live and express themselves through the arts until their eighties and even nineties. He cites Grandma Moses, Goethe, Richard Strauss, Verdi, Schuetz and Sibelius as practising their arts until the end (1997, p. 81).

Also interested in creativity, neuroscientist Norman Doidge (2007) cites Frank Lloyd-Wright as designing the Guggenheim Museum in his 90s and Benjamin Franklin inventing bi-focal spectacles at 78. He tells us: "When Pablo Casals, the cellist, was 91 years old, he was approached by a student who asked, 'Master, why do you continue to practice?' Casals replied, 'Because I am making progress'" (Doidge, 2007, p. 258).

John Zeisel, president and co-founder of Hearthstone Alzheimer Care and Hearthstone Alzheimer's Foundation, USA (2009), is also passionate about artistic as well as non-pharmacologic ways of treating Alzheimer's disease (AD). He believes that by understanding music and art through touch and facial expressions, people with severe dementia show that they are highly creative and emotionally intelligent. By harnessing these qualities and using techniques such as gallery visiting to view well-known and easily recognisable paintings, he believes it is possible to increase people's QoL, as well as their connection to others and to the world (Zeisel, personal communication, June 15, 2010). In the intervening 10 years since my conversation with John Zeisel, there have been many global initiatives in the world's cities and art galleries to bring the elderly into contact with visual art. For example, The Artz Artists for Alzheimer's program in the USA (Hearthstone Artz "I'm Still Here" Foundation, 2019) assists in bringing "emotional memory" alive and keeping cognitive functioning at a balanced level in group visits to the Museum of Modern Art in New York City. The National Gallery of Australia's Art and Dementia Program is using cortisol biomarkers to investigate the health and wellbeing of participants. Post-program self-reported indicators of depression have decreased, and memory and verbal ability have improved. When treated with respect and dignity, participants' own memories and experience have allowed them to engage with the art works they viewed (D'Cunha, 2019). These gallery visiting initiatives have emerged from the Hearthstone Foundation's pioneering work.

Today, neuroscience is playing an ever more important role in arts therapies. However, the neurological and art therapy literature express the connection between art making and the brain very differently. Safar and Press (2018) bring these two together in an attempt to integrate them, relating the production of art works to neurological illness, such that simultaneously, dynamic therapeutic progress can occur with an understanding of dementia from the point of view of neurology. The decline in her capacity to make art is documented by them in a client who is also an experienced artist. Connecting lines to one another, for example, becomes more difficult and the client expresses this as "trying to find the magic line" (p. 98). The application of an awareness of the interactions of various parts of the brain with art production can assist the therapist to understand how the client can be affected from a psychological point of view and adjust the therapy correspondingly. Neuroscience-informed art psychotherapy can achieve outcomes that would not have been possible with talking therapy on its own.

Something comparable can happen when people with dementia join a choir or listen to music. Robertson-Gillam (2014) used brain imaging when she investigated the possibility of reducing social isolation and depressive symptoms in people with dementia in her choir therapy program (CTP). She states:

> The CTP is effective as an adjunct intervention for reducing major depression in mid to later life. Further research should assess each segment of the program as well as compare the CTP with other creative arts programs for reducing symptoms of major depression in mid to later life.
>
> (2014, p. xv)

Oliver Sacks, in *Musicophilia*, explores the very human engagement with, and love of, music and its ability to help us to "respond powerfully and specifically to music. Some of these patients have widespread cortical problems, whether from strokes or Alzheimer's or other causes of dementia" (Sacks, 2007, p. xiii). Sacks explains how music can affect us with particular intensity, where we experience comfort and grief simultaneously (2007). His approach has taught us about an important healing approach to grief. We cannot avoid the bleak truths of grieving; however, with the re-membering of the losses comes an unlooked-for benefit – a certain sense of healing that we know we can return to whenever we return to the old memory. These questions will be dealt with further in Chapter 8.

The question of psychotherapy, sometimes an ideal way to deal with grief, has been given a mixed response with elderly people in the available theoretical literature on the subject. However, Krishna et al. (2011) undertook a systematic review of six articles which met their quantitative ratings on the efficacy of group psychotherapy on older adults with depression, based on previous quantitative meta-analyses. They eliminated studies which were qualitative only and included patients using other therapies or who were experiencing other primary mental illnesses such as psychosis or a diagnosis of alcohol or drug dependence. Using a rating scale to extract data from each study, they found that there was a case for the effectiveness of such treatments. In 2009, Cheston and Jones compared psychoeducational interventions and psychotherapy in people with Alzheimer's or similar types of dementia. Their study provides evidence to suggest that in a 10-week course of exploratory group work, "psychotherapy can decrease levels of depression for people with dementia at a mild level of cognitive impairment" (2009, p. 424). The authors found that further research would be necessary to determine similar results in the psychoeducation group.

In a group analytical study of psychotherapy with people experiencing dementia, Hadar (2018) comments on an article written with a focus on fighting ageism by Perren and Richardson (2018). She highlights the fact that the facilitators struggled to introduce group psychotherapy for elderly people with dementia in a hospital where there was a bias against this mode of therapy and where the busy staff disrespectfully "popped in" to see what was happening in the group meetings, considering them pointless. The facilitators, who were acknowledging their own ageism, felt isolated within the institution. In the wider therapeutic structure of the hospital, the group was judged to be valueless and was ignored and forgotten. Despite the dismissive attitude of the other staff, Perren and Richardson's investigation found there was a sense of "togetherness and belonging; normality and safety and greater freedom to express emotion" than the control group (2018, p. 15). Hadar asks the question, "What should our attitude be towards psychotherapy with people who are not going to recover—those whose psychological and physical trajectory are deteriorating, not improving?" (2018, p. 105). She finds that the difficult work that relatively inexperienced facilitators/researchers were doing with their groups (comparing a psychotherapy group with a psychosocial one) had an important relevance here. By means of answering the question, she uses the words of validation therapist Naomi Feil, who says: "When people are very old and deteriorating, and no one enters their world, and they are just sitting, they will withdraw inward more and more, and their desperate need for connection is all inside" (cited by Hadar, p. 105). Feil's words stand as a confirmation of the need for psychotherapy for the elderly, whether or not they have dementia.

A further reason for psychotherapy is the participants' ability to share with others some of the more scary and isolating aspects of dementia. It also presents the opportunity to deal with some emotionally charged feelings which emerge from the experience so that they can be processed rather than suppressed (Cheston et al., 2003). There is some evidence of behavioural and psychological symptoms of dementia (BPSD) resulting from some of the fear and loneliness referred to above being reduced by short-term psychotherapy

(Ericson & Eriksson, 2013). Studies of psychotherapeutic treatment of people with dementia are becoming rarer (Linnemann & Fellgiebel, 2017), and yet psychotherapy can be very effective, especially in the early stages of dementia.

Hadar and Feil's attitudes to psychotherapy with the elderly, and especially people with dementia, come close to arts therapists' views on their psychotherapeutic work with them. Spalding and Khalsa (2010) write about humanistic and transpersonal approaches to psychotherapy with people with dementia. Their research is focused on the experience of psychotherapy interns when applying such approaches to their relationships with elderly clients rather than the pharmacology model of care. The investigation uses a phenomenological method known as the Boyatzis qualitative thematic analysis method to code the interview transcripts. Boyatzis (1998) focused on addressing the paucity of qualitative research related to the nuanced aspects of lived experience of dementia. Themes are developed and organised as in grounded theory. In their literature review of studies of mainstream approaches and attitudes to such people, Spalding and Khalsa note the following:

> What is typically diagnosed as pathology may in fact be an individual's need to process, prepare, rehearse, or repair, emphasising healing and growth over maintenance and comfort. Such organic unfolding of symptoms is likely to be inhibited by excessive medication, often the prescribed norm for clinical patients. Well-intentioned attempts to control and minimize symptoms can both antagonise and undermine the clients' and therapists' recognition of an underlying coherence and meaning to the various psychological, emotional, physical, and possibly spiritual signals that comprise the diverse experience of dementia.
>
> (2010, p. 144)

Once their interviews were coded and analysed, it was found that the intern trainee therapists involved in their study – the participants – all believed in a probable subjective significance and essential value to their clients' dementia experience, separate from and disassociated with loss and decline. Most claimed that this meaning could be present and secure in the therapist's "holding" role when there were memory lapses on the part of participants. Indeed, many of the interviewees reported that simply bestowing a value on the onset and progression of dementia could lead to a more potent co-investigation of the participants' experience (Spalding & Khalsa, 2010). Their views fit well with Tornstam's (1993, 2005) expansion of self in the elderly as well as O'Neil and O'Neil's (1990) "renewal and resurgence of creative forces" (pp. 226–227). This may include the value of any sadness being recognised and acknowledged as part of the human condition and constellation of feelings at any stage. As such, when sadness occurs, there is an intimate and personal value in being witnessed by the therapist and other group participants in the dramatherapy process.

These seeds of hope for the elderly and people who have dementia are explored in the following chapter, where the diagnosis of dementia is discussed, as well as the lived experience of those who live their lives under its shadow.

References

Australian Broadcasting Commission. (2017). Old people's home for four-year-olds [Video]. Available from https://iview.abc.net.au › show › old-people-s-home-for-four-year-olds

Boyatzis, R. (1998). *Transforming qualitative information: Thematic analysis and code development*. Sage.

Buber, M. (1965). *I and Thou*. T. & T. Clark.

Cheston, R., Jones, K., & Gilliard, J. (2003). Group psychotherapy and people with dementia. *Aging and Mental Health*, 7(6), 452–461.

Cheston, R., & Jones, R. (2009). A small-scale study comparing the impact of psycho-education and exploratory psychotherapy groups on newcomers to a group for people with dementia. *Aging and Mental Health*, 13(3), 420–425.

D'Cunha, N. (2019). Psychophysiological responses of people living with dementia after an art gallery intervention: An exploratory study. *Journal of Alzheimer's Disease*, 72(2), 549–562.

Dementia Australia. (2021). Progression of dementia. Retrieved October 28, 2021, from https://www.dementia.org.au/about-dementia/whatisdementia/progression-of-dementia

Doidge, N. (2007). *The brain that changes itself*. Scribe.

Ericson, A., & Eriksson, S. (2013). Intensive short-term dynamic psychotherapy in dementia: A pilot study. *International Journal of Geriatric Psychiatry*, 28(8), 877–879.

Erikson, E. H. (1963). *Childhood and society*. W. W. Norton.

Erikson, E. H. (1997). *The life cycle completed*. Extended version by J. M. Erikson. W. W. Norton & Co., Inc.

Erikson, E. H., Erikson, J. M., & Kivnick, H. Q. (1989). *Vital involvement in old age*. W. W. Norton & Co., Inc.

Freud, S. (1905). *On psychotherapy*. Reprinted (1953–74) in *Standard edition of the complete works of Sigmund Freud* (trans. & ed. J. Strachey; Vol. 7). Hogarth Press.

Gordon-Flower, M. (2020). *Arts therapies with people with physical disabilities*. Jessica Kingsley.

Hadar, B. (2018). Response to "Everybody needs a group: A qualitative study looking at therapists' views of the role of psychotherapy groups in working with older people with dementia and complex needs". *Group Analysis*, 51(1), 102–109.

Hearthstone Artz "I'm still here" Foundation. (2019). "Artz artists for Alzheimers" program. Retrieved November 18, 2019, from http://www.programsforelderly.com/memory-artz-artists-for-alzheimers.php

Jaaniste, E. J. (2013). *Pulled through a hedge backwards: Improving the quality of life of people with dementia through dramatherapy* [Unpublished PhD Thesis]. University of Western Sydney.

Jaaniste, J. (2016). Lifestage and human development in dramatherapy with people who have dementia. In C. Holmwood & S. Jennings (Eds.), *Routledge international handbook of dramatherapy*. Routledge.

Jung, C. J. (1991). *The structure and dynamics of the psyche* (2nd ed.). Princeton University Press.

Krishna, M., Jauhari, A., Lepping, P., Turner, J., & Krishnamoorthy, A. (2011). Is group psychotherapy effective in older adults with depression? A systematic review. *International Journal of Geriatric Psychiatry, 26*(4), 331–340.

Lievegoed, B. (1997). *Phases: The spiritual rhythms in adult life.* Sophia Books.

Linnemann, A., & Fellgiebel, A. (2017). Psychotherapie bei leichter kognitiver Beeinträchtigung und Demenz. *Der Nervenarzt, 88*(11), 1240–1245.

Malone, J. C., Liu, S. R., Vaillant, G. E., Rentz, G. M., & Waldinger, R. A. (2016). Midlife Ericksonian psychological development: Setting the stage for late-life cognitive and emotional health. *Developmental Psychology, 52*(3), 496–508.

Morrison, R., & Siu, A. (2000). Survival in end-stage dementia following acute illness. *Journal of the American Medical Association, 284*(1), 47–52.

O'Neil, G., & O'Neil, G. (1990). *The human life.* Mercury Press.

Perren, S., & Richardson, T. (2018). Everybody needs a group: A qualitative study looking at therapists' views of the role of psychotherapy groups in working with older people with dementia and complex needs. *Group Analysis, 51*(1), 3–17.

Prétat, J. (1994). *Coming to age: The croning years and late-life transformation.* Inner City Books.

Robertson-Gillam, K. (2014). *Reducing major depression in mid to later life with a choir therapy program: A mixed methods study* [Doctoral dissertation, University of Western Sydney (Australia)]. ProQuest Dissertations Publishing.

Sacks, O. (2007). *Musicophilia.* Vintage Books.

Safar, L. T., & Press, D. Z. (2018). Art and the brain: Effects of dementia on art production in art therapy. *Journal of the American Art Therapy Association, 28*(3), 96–103.

Shakespeare, W. (1876). *The dramatic works of William Shakespeare* (T. Campbell, Ed.). George Routledge & Sons.

Skropeta, C. M., Colvin, A., & Sladen, S. (2014). An evaluative study of the benefits of participating in intergenerational playgroups in aged care for older people. Retrieved December 6, 2019, from www.biomedcentral.com/1471-2318/14/109

Spalding, M., & Khalsa, P. (2010). Aging matters: Humanistic and transpersonal approaches to psychotherapy with elders with dementia. *Journal of Humanistic Psychology, 50*(2), 142–174.

Teater, B. (2016). Intergenerational programs to promote active aging: The experiences and perspectives of older adults. *Activities, Adaptation and Aging, 40*(1), 1–19.

Tornstam, L. (1993). Gerotranscendence: The contemplative dimension of aging. *Journal of Aging Studies, 11*(2), 143–154.

Tornstam, L. (2005). *Gerotranscendence: A developmental theory of positive aging.* Springer.

Weisberg, N., & Wilder, R. (2001). *Expressive arts with elders* (2nd ed.). Jessica Kingsley.

Zeisel, J. (2009). *I'm still here.* Penguin Books Ltd.

Chapter 2

What is it like to have dementia?

In a chapter I wrote for a collection of essays on dementia and creativity (Jaaniste, 2011), I contributed the following anecdotal material from an early experience of working with the elderly. My long-held belief since childhood in the dignity and imaginative capacity of people with dementia shaped my response:

> My first experience of improvisation and dementia came as a young mother in her early thirties, working night shifts, with no knowledge of dramatherapy, as a nursing assistant in a home for elderly people. Mavis, who had dementia, would come downstairs in the middle of the night, informing her care worker that she could not return to bed, because her husband was still away and the roast dinner was ready. Up to the bedroom we would go, and I would ask Mavis to look out of the window for her husband Bob while I helped to "prod the roast", and then got her to "help set the table". When everything was ready, and she was sure she could hear Bob's footsteps on the stairs, she would get back into bed. Improvisation had solved the midnight wandering.
>
> (Jaaniste, 2011)

I learned from Mavis that if I respected the world of memory that she inhabited that evening as if it were in the present moment, we could find a way to resolve her immediate pain, which poignantly re-enacts an ongoing sense of loss. My clients in acute and community mental health over the past 24 years have also taught me a great deal – they have trained me, showing me the way to empathise with their deep suffering and revealing the "mad person" inside me. I have no experience of the depths of severe depression; however, coming from a family where there is an over-supply of mental illness and losing a sister through suicide, grief has taught me many lessons. This learning has led me joyfully into the therapeutic work with people who are elderly, whose bodies are failing them and whose friends have died (Jaaniste, 2013).

DOI: 10.4324/9781003186328-2

According to the Diagnostic and Statistical Manual of Mental Disorders (American Psychiatric Association, 2013), dementia is the overarching term for a number of conditions of a neurological nature. The primary symptom is a reduction in the way the brain operates due to physical alterations, not to be confused with mental illness (American Psychiatric Association, 2013). It is classified as a neurocognitive disorder (NCD):

- if the cognitive deficits interfere with independence
- if they do not occur exclusively in the context of a delirium
- if they are not significantly attributable to another mental disorder such as major depressive disorder and schizophrenia
- if there is evidence of substantial cognitive decline from a previous level of performance in one or more of the domains listed below:
- **Complex attention** – involves sustained attention, divided attention, selective attention and information processing speed
  Warning signs – Patient has increased difficulty in environments with multiple stimuli (TV, radio, conversation). Has difficulty holding new information in mind (recalling phone numbers or addresses just given or reporting what was just said).
- **Executive ability** – involves planning, decision making, working memory, responding to feedback, error correction, overriding habits and mental flexibility
  Warning signs – Patient is unable to perform both familiar and complex tasks and projects (at work and at home). Needs to rely on others to plan instrumental activities of daily living or make decisions. Has problems with abstract thinking, displays loss of initiative as well as poor/decreased judgement.
- **Learning and memory** – involves immediate memory, recent memory (free recall, cued recall and recognition memory) and long-term memory
  Warning signs – Patient repeats self in conversation, often with the same conversation. Cannot keep track of short list of items when shopping or of plans for the day. Requires frequent reminders to orient task at hand, confusion about time and place, and repetitive behaviour.
- **Language** – involves expressive language (naming, fluency, grammar and syntax) and receptive language
  Warning signs – Patient has significant difficulties with expressive or receptive language. Often uses general terms such as "that thing" and "you know what I mean". With severe impairment may not recall names of closer friends and family.
- **Perceptual – Motor – Visual perception, praxis** – involves picking up the telephone, handwriting, using a fork/spoon
  Warning signs – Patient has significant difficulties with previously familiar activities (using tools or driving a motor vehicle) and navigating in familiar environments.

- **Social cognition** – involves recognition of emotions and behavioural regulation, social appropriateness in terms of dress, grooming and topics of conversation
  Warning signs – Patient may have changes in behaviour (shows insensitivity to social standards, or make decisions without regard to safety). Patient usually has little insight into these changes. Becomes socially withdrawn or isolated (American Psychiatric Association, 2013).

In NCD, a well-known variety of which is Alzheimer's disease (AD), brain atrophy and symptoms of cell degeneration can be detected microscopically (Kitwood, 1997) and now of course, tomography is used, with computed tomography (CT) scans and magnetic resonance imaging (MRIs). The change in the DSM-5 has been made to facilitate a more accurate diagnosis, of mild NCD and major NCD, followed by the different sub-types of the causes of NCD, such as Alzheimer's, Huntington's or HIV infection. Although the threshold between mild and major NCD is inherently arbitrary, the two levels of impairment are considered separately for consistency with other fields of medicine and to capture the care needs of people living with NCD (Dementia Australia, Q&A 11, 2022, pp. 1–2). In my view, the previous differentiation between mild, moderate and severe dementia made it much easier to capture the stages of dementia and the trajectory taken by the disease over time. The 2013 changes may also be confusing to carers whose family members have had dementia for a very long time, when there is less differentiation than before.

Signs of degeneration are most often seen in plaque deposits and neurofibrillary tangles found through tomography or autopsy. Kitwood (1997) and Power (2011; 2017) describe a traditional view of dementia as one that emphasises loss and deficits, encouraging approaches to care that are institutional and based on disease (as in the deficits of brain function described above in the DSM-5 definition). Referring to the regrettable assessment of people with dementia by their inabilities, rather than their strengths, Power cites the widely used mini-mental status examination (MMSE) (Folstein et al., 1975), where there is a litany of discrete tasks to be performed: "Can you spell 'world' backwards? Can you remember three objects after five minutes? Can you copy a figure of two intersecting pentagrams?" (2011, p. x). Surely, these kinds of tasks are extraordinarily difficult for many people who are not experiencing problems of the kind associated with dementia, let alone for people for whom English is not their first language in an English-speaking country. Carnero-Pardo (2014) believes the MMSE should be honourably retired, and that an alternative that is "less time-consuming user-friendly and free of charge, can be applied to all individuals and yield more equitable outcomes" (Carnero-Pardo, 2014, p. 473). It seems appropriate to raise the question of how relevant these tasks are, and to ask who the results are for – the medical profession, the carer or actually the person with dementia who is being diagnosed.

Regardless of often cited and documented validity and reliability, there is a poignant question about the relevance of the questions Power (2011) mentions for the daily lives of the people being diagnosed. As it is, there is a need for cultural adaptation of the measure for people who live in low to middle-income countries, as many believe there is an educational bias in the scale (Bertolucci et al., 1994; Chaves, 2014; Tiwiri et al., 2009). There appears to be general agreement that the severe mini-mental state examination (SMMSE) (Harrell et al., 2000) is a simpler measure for diagnosing dementia in people with low levels of education (Chaves, 2014; Wajeman & Bertolucci, 2006).

The above tests seem to take less time for the diagnostician than anything more suited to the person who needs them. The all-important time factor also brings stress into facilities for the aged, whereas our ageing population deserve the respect due to them and their slower-paced ways. A more appropriate and certainly more humane way of going about diagnosis seems to be neuropsychological testing, which takes longer, but can be carried out over more than one visit. This is usually completed by a psychologist who has been trained in dementia and other disorders of mental functioning. A range of tests are given, depending on the educational level and cognitive ability of the client. The measures could include drawing, reproducing figures presented to the client, as well as other tests of reasoning and comprehension (Dementia Australia, Q&A 10, 2022, p. 4). This might help to overcome what is actually a human rights issue.

There are problems with the diagnosis of dementia, especially where there are pre-existing or exacerbating health problems. Byers and Yaffe (2011) indicate that patients experiencing depression may have a kind of "pseudodementia" which is problematic and requires careful diagnosis. They recommend that a life course approach be taken to a study of depression and dementia. "Earlier-life depression has been shown to be an important risk factor for dementia, but whether it is a true risk factor for development of dementia or whether a third factor causes depression and dementia is still unknown" (Byers & Yaffe, 2011, p. 329). Yaffe et al. (2010) were also among the first to discover that veterans of war who had post-traumatic stress disorder (PTSD) were more likely than those in the rest of the community to acquire early dementia (see Chapter 7). They say that research participants were diagnosed according to the WHO International Classification of Diseases 9 (ICD-9), so that we can infer that they were diagnosed with the MMSE. Shively et al. (2013) found from epidemiological studies that traumatic brain injury (TBI), where damage is sustained in early to mid-life, is an indicator of increased risk of dementia in later life. The rates of this risk were found to be two to four times those of the general population. Tomography, or MRI scans, were the means of diagnosis of the dementia.

At a time when the World Health Organization (WHO) is informing us of an ever-rising figure of 55 million people around the world with dementia (2021), it is important that we recognise the humanity of such people and embrace alternatives to a dominant "disease narrative". Power, writing of the "hidden disability caused by disenfranchising care" (Adams & Lee, 2011, p. xiii) makes the following claim for dementia and creative engagement, moving the discourse to a new area of creativity: "... the excess disability (is) caused by a care approach that positions, disempowers, isolates and overmedicates the person" (p. x). In 2017 Richard Taylor stated in his introduction to Power's book that we position people as lacking capability and research disregards the "lived experience of people with dementia: "Creative engagement enables us to remove much of this excess disability, and people's own experience informs new abilities thought to be long lost to their illness" (Power, 2017, p. xiv). Kontos and Martin's (2013) contribution has also been part of a movement towards a greater recognition of the way that human beings need to be seen as embodied creatures, and this has "broadened and enriched the discourse on selfhood and memory in dementia" (Kontos & Martin, 2013, p. 289).

Power goes on to describe how the "biomedical approach to dementia" (Adams & Lee, 2011, p. x) encourages us to set up environments (and, I would add, form attitudes) which are more appropriate to the needs of the care force or family carers than to individuals living with the diagnosis. If we can alter our focus from a one-size-fits-all model to a more holistic one, we are more likely to understand the worldview of the person with dementia (2011). In 2013, in speaking about the *Spark of Life* program for the elderly in Western Australia, he advised:

> Many people living with dementia experience different types of distress. I think this is because it is more difficult for them to maintain a sense of wellbeing when they are cognitively challenged. The traditional view is that this is due to damaged brain cells, which is why we often reach for medications. But the truth is that there are all of these underlying emotional needs that are often poorly identified and recognised by the traditional approach.
>
> (Power, 2013)

With regard to medications, an experience of creative engagement such as dramatherapy could be a valid substitution for medication, especially where a person is experiencing "sundowning". This is a term for restless moving around, a sense of disquiet and anxiety or confusion in people with dementia that can occur in the late afternoon simultaneously with caregivers needing a break. People experiencing such distressing episodes are often medicated.

The Mayo Clinic suggests it can occur in facilities where there is a lack of structured activity in the afternoon (Graff-Radford, 2020), although more research needs to be done in the area.

In the light of the above authors' open-minded approaches to development at the end of life, an overview of developmental theories and their application to later stages of life are introduced here. They are intended to present questions for the dramatherapist and others working with people with dementia. How far do we apply these stages, and how do they help a participant understand the meaning of their existence up to this point?

Symptom of dementia	Attribute of normal later developmental life stage
Lack of consistent information retention	Deterioration of the ability to concentrate
Decreased problem-solving ability	Greater reliance on others to help make decisions
Short-term memory loss	Greater reliance on list-writing and reminders
Loss of fine motor skills	Difficulty in threading needles and using some tools
Social withdrawal, isolation	Enjoyment in sitting quietly
Involved in past memories	Reflection on past life events
A feeling of closeness to lost loved ones	Strong memories of lost loved ones

How does dramatherapy help people who are elderly, who have dementia? I believe it has a healing quality which speaks to the soul of people in their later life stages. By the soul is meant the means by which we link experiences to our own being, through which we feel pleasure and displeasure, desire and aversion, joy and sorrow, in relation to them (Steiner, 1993, p. 18). Steiner writes of denial of the soul as trying to run away from it: "a desire to run away from one's own soul. This, however, represents an impossibility. One must remain with oneself" (Steiner, 1985, p. 29). Dramatherapy enables us to stay within our soul, through our imagination and creativity. The concept of soul, although sometimes unfashionable, is in fact extremely helpful in alerting people to their own actual presence. Auguste D, the very first patient with dementia of Dr Alois Alzheimer, after whom AD is named, said in 1901, "So to speak, I lost myself" (Yang et. al., 2016). This statement seems to be a sign that Auguste D knows she has a self to lose. Sadly, her statement appears to have resulted in encouraging a view of dementia as a "loss of self and a changing identity" and people with the diagnosis as "the other" (Naue & Kroll, 2008, p. 26).

For many of our well-known Australians, dementia has come to them later in life and they have written or been interviewed on its effects for their lives. Anne Deveson was a much-loved Australian broadcaster, writer, filmmaker and social commentator, who reached out to those who had lost young people through suicide and herself survived huge challenges through resilience. She spoke to Fenella Souter in 2015, telling her that it was necessary to move forward past the disease, as she was not identified by dementia. Souter reports, in Deveson's words, that she has struggled not to be overtaken by the illness,

> ... with its rounds of appointments, care arrangements, being bossed about and so on. Even if your brain goes, you can still enjoy the sky and the sun and the trees and all sorts of things, but it takes a while to get to that part.
>
> (Souter, 2015, p. 19)

Christine Bryden was a top civil servant before she was diagnosed with dementia much younger, at the age of 46. She spent the next few years writing and lobbying for greater understanding and dignity for people with dementia, telling readers of her experience of the disease. Her second book, *Dancing with dementia*, describes her difficulties with loss of memory and doing simple tasks. She writes about each person's journey:

> ... deep into the core of their spirit, away from the complex cognitive outer layer that once defined them, through the jumble and tangle of emotions created through their life experiences, into the centre of their being, into what truly gives them meaning in life. Many of us seek earnestly for this sense of the present time, the sense of 'now', of how to live each moment and treasure it as if it were the only experience to look at and to wonder at.
>
> (Bryden, 2005, p. 11)

"Dramatherapy can help with keeping people in the present moment", as Sally Bailey, American drama therapist attests. "People who are not always 'with it' in reality still know when they are pretending" (Garrett, 2006, para. 3).

These people have made it easier for the public to understand that dementia is not all challenge and difficulty, although for some, it may seem that way for family members. Popular journalist, Mike Carlton, writing in a Sydney local newspaper in 2012, entitled his column "Oh for a glimpse of the Mum I knew". He describes how much his mother had changed as the disease progressed. She had been a keen gardener and loved knitting and now her dementia had made her afraid even to turn on the television. Her family needed to remove her phone ...

> ... because she was running up huge bills making the same call to say the same anxious thing to the same person, every half hour. Her days and nights are spent lying on a bed in a small, beige room, staring at the walls and waiting to die.
>
> (Carlton, 2012, p. 16)

As I write, the Royal Commission into Aged Care is taking place in Australia. Their Quality and Safety Interim Report records serious failures in the aged care system that have unfortunately not been detailed as breaches of human rights (Cheu, 2019). Cheu documents the views of a Professor of Gerontology speaking to delegates at a concurrent conference about the Royal Commission: "It is striking how little reference the report makes to human rights. Even as it details and denounces a litany of practices that are human rights violations that result from the failure of the system" (Byrne, as cited in Cheu, 2019). This report calls into question situations like that of Mike Carlton's mother "staring at the walls and waiting to die". If person-centred care (Kitwood, 1997) were practised throughout the system, it is more likely that the arts therapies would be available to people like her, and her human rights would be intact, at least for creative therapy sessions. This would be the case even in a country like Australia which has no actual Bill of Rights, and must therefore rely on the integrity of government institutions and non-government organisations (NGOs) to assist people with dementia to treat clients with respect and provide opportunities for good quality of life (QoL). Even in severe dementia where people are finding it hard to retrieve words, they can usually still move and dramatherapy can assist with their QoL. The Royal Commission is investigating over-medication, which could easily be replaced by low-cost dance movement or dramatherapy.

McKeith and Cummings (2005) state, in their phenomenological review and analysis of the various types of dementia, that behavioural and psychological symptoms of dementia (BPSD) have generally been thought to be of secondary importance to areas of physical function. There is evidence, however, suggesting that certain behaviours are important determinants of patients' distress, carer burden and outcomes in dementia. Though the authors admit that pharmacological management is a commonly used option, it is often limited in its effects and can be associated with a substantial risk of side effects. They recommend non-pharmacological interventions and include behavioural therapies, systematic changes of the care environment, exercise and music instead. Physical movement and embodiment of meaning will be covered in more detail in the session below, where it is shown, using a developmental paradigm, that people who have severe dementia can express themselves robustly through sound and movement.

A session entitled Planting seeds was the fifth in a series of 16 weekly sessions. The symbolic activity of the planting was intended to show that even though the participants had been diagnosed with dementia, they had planted seeds in their lives which had flourished and would go on growing, as their own resilience also had the chance to do. The movement work supported this aspect of the session.

Initial discussion and warm-ups

The session started with the usual chat about who was there and who was missing. I brought up the title of the session and with it the thought that a diagnosis of dementia should not get in the way of growth. I asked whether anyone ever had the experience of getting a diagnosis of Alzheimer's or dementia and then wondered what that might mean for the rest of their lives. Neil immediately said he had, and Peter said he had definitely asked himself this question. So I asked Neil to speak first. He said:

> Well, just that it was as – it was just like that. The diagnosis. I'm not saying that there wasn't, um, yeah, there was, not treatment, um, tests, I suppose. Yeah, so there were tests. But, um, yeah, it still came as a very harsh thing.

When I questioned the word "harsh", he said: "Mmm … as if, you know, fell off the side of a building".

There was a silence in the room for a few moments as everyone took this in. Then I agreed that it was harsh and asked him what his fears or thoughts for his life might have been. Neil said:

> There were more than fears. There are realities. Ah, we were just talking about driving, and, um, it came down like that. It wasn't, you know, maybe you can drive for another year. It wasn't like that. The – I forget the title – the doctor, well, not a – the doctor said don't drive. So that's like a – it wasn't the only thing. That was a problem but, um, that became the problem.

Then it was Peter's turn to speak:

> … things happened to me, just like you, relative to driving. And, um, I, um, actually came to the conclusion when I'm still driving and still had a license that I wasn't safe. Um, and that because I was sort of getting muddled up with things which was – and it was made worse by the fact that the government was busy changing everything. So you had to, um, sort of – you could – you did just come out of the drive and drive off like that. You had to come out of, of the other thing and check whether it was Tuesday, Wednesday, Thursday, Friday, Saturday and then you had to sort of work out whether it was something that you, um, were allowed to do or not allowed to do and all that type of … And they were – and they sort of, um, gummed up the actual action of it and I decided I wasn't safe to drive.

Leanne felt "corralled" – there was definitely a sense in which the driving represented independence for her and people felt controlled by the ruling.

This was closer to Mike Carlton's Mum lying in a "small, beige room". However, when I asked David how he reacted when he was told he had dementia, he said: "I don't know – I've got dementia" at which there was plenty of laughter. He said later on that he felt frustrated because of his inability to play sport and perform handyman jobs around the house.

Because of the initial conversation about the diagnosis, there was a sense of being trapped, as evidenced by Leanne's comment and Paul's comments about the cold ("I've got my socks on underneath" and "it either comes out warm or cold"). We had been sitting for a while, so the warm-ups took the form of walking around the room leading with various body parts, and then changed to passing a facial expression around the circle. There were no comments at all about the first warm-up, as people tried with varying degrees of success to lead with a particular part of their body, demonstrated by myself and the staff members. However, once participants had an explanation of mirroring, there was a great deal of laughter and camaraderie in the second, in the engagement with and mirroring of twisted and forced facial expressions. This was a preparation for "becoming" different kinds of plants and trees, in tune with the theme of growth. As dramatherapist Nisha Sajnani said in her speech launching the Creative Arts Therapies Research Unit at Melbourne University (2016) about her experience moving from theatre to dramatherapy: "Difficult topics were easier to talk about when we could turn them into a physical tableau or enactment". Also, as Langley (2006) points out, memory activation is important in games and warm-ups with people with dementia.

Mirroring, sculpture and self-sculpture are well-known techniques in psychodrama and dramatherapy (Blatner, 1988; Emunah, 1994). These techniques are used in family therapy where typically they reveal, through their positioning of clients with others in a group, a representation of their family of origin (Emunah, 1994). Participants are often physically manoeuvred by another, either from the family or by a director within the situational psychodrama. Here, however, the sculpted position is chosen by the participants themselves as their favourite tree, or as themselves in achievement mode, mirroring with the help of the therapist or a support person in the group. The partner in the dyad is there to take up the other's position and mirror the body sculpt back to the participant, so they have an idea of how they looked in the sculpt. In the work that follows, the sculpting of trees was used, not only to tune in with the theme of growth but also to prepare participants for a further sculpt of a biographical nature which would influence their choice of positioning for a collaborative dance movement. Thus there may be a subtle sense of the self-revelatory position which is often part of the family therapy or psychodrama model; however, the main intentional thrust is to have participants cooperate in an individual gesture that belongs to their lived experience, which will then be shared with others in a collaborative dance. The participant is using their body to represent a high point in their life experience.

Participants were asked what kind of tree they would prefer to sculpt and were assisted with their body formations to become the tree of their choice. Once these "trees" were performed for the others, they were asked to walk around and look for cards placed on the floor, with words about growth on them, such as "rising", "green", "organic" and "growing". There were blank cards there too, which the participants could write on, which they did, with words such as: "sunrise", "ageing", "spreading – shrinking", "extending", "looking forward" and "strength". Ben, who generally used group opportunities to handwrite while others were painting or drawing, filled his card: "Growth of local flowers; well in stock; renewal of flowers; in the best of districts". It seemed, from a metaphorical viewpoint, that there was some resilience already happening and his language suggested participant growth in the group environment. They were then asked to take a partner and talk to them about symbolic seeds they had planted in their lives, such as David as a Bondi lifesaver teaching people how to do surf rescue, and Paul, an architect teaching creativity in building design. Once participant A had decided on an appropriate sculpt with their partner, we helped them to find a body position which represented their achievement and helped their partner B to copy it and mirror it back to them. A would then take the pose up again and perform it to B. They would then change roles, and it would be B's turn to take their own individual pose, and the process would be repeated for them. Once this was achieved, participants were then asked to form a group, together with staff and student supporters, to form a dance out of these sculpts. Music came through the i-pod, and everyone danced in a group, sharing their sculpts as they created a moving synthesis of their work.

It was surprising for me to see these elderly people moving to the music and discovering one another's movements. It was the climax of an embodiment process. Richard Coaten describes the process of hand movements which extend their flow into a fuller embodiment:

> The most important aspect of this experiential work [...] is to remember to take pleasure in it all. If it can remain pleasurable, observed 'well-being' will have increased and 'ill-being' decreased. Together, you will have played and danced in embodied ways that truly offer hope in going by way of the body in dementia care, when words are not enough.
>
> (Coaten, 2011, p. 88)

When we returned to our places in the circle, Ben started talking about being at a race track, which reminded me that perhaps we had gone too quickly for him in the series of activities that had happened since he came in that morning. Other than this, as experienced by Coaten above, there was very little contribution to the reflection on the exercises which were performed in the here-and-now, other than smiles and facial expressions of pleasure. The pots of earth and crocus bulbs were then introduced – each pot had the name of one of the participants attached to it. They were given instructions on how deeply they should plant them, and asked to give their plant a message as they were embedded. Ben gave his message: "It'll be very hard – very hard for you to be coming up". Perhaps the "race" through the previous activities had affected his mood. David was next; he said, "Grow tall and straight". Neil said, "Branch out" and Leanne said, "Grow". Each time someone spoke to their plant, the other participants repeated their message back to them. At first, Paul said he would not speak to the plant, but then he changed his mind. As a literary person who knew several languages, he said, "honi soit qui mal y pense" or in other words, "Shame come to him who thinks badly of it". They were then asked what they were taking away from the group, as it was coming to an end. Paul said, "Some good ideas"; David: "Very pleasant planting the bulb"; Ben: "It was easy and on top of some material and it should work for us. Thank you"; Leanne: "I hope that my plant will grow" and Neil: "Early release". It should be noted that Neil was still at the stage where he was not sure if he really wanted to be there at all and may have been ready to see his carer come in and accompany him home. However, when he spoke much later at the final and 16th session, he said:

> I made connections through the program. Even simple things like the songs. I love those. And it was … the program here. It was very simple things like that. You know, I'd be sad if I would go today and not have that.

A session which had begun with the hard realisation of receiving a dementia diagnosis with its inevitable loss of independence ended with a sense that the possibility for growth and resilience was still there.

References

American Psychiatric Association. (2013). *Diagnostic and statistical manual of mental disorder* (5th ed.). Washington D.C.

Bertolucci, P. H. F., Brucki, S. M. D., Campacci, S. R., & Juliano, Y. (1994). The mini-mental state examination in an outpatient population: Influence of literacy. *Arquivos Neuropsiquiatria, 52*(1), 1–7.

Blatner, A. (1988). *Foundations of psychodrama: History, theory and practice* (3rd ed.). Springer Publishing.

Bryden, C. (2005). *Dancing with dementia*. Jessica Kingsley Press.

Byers, A., & Yaffe, C. (2011). Depression and risk of developing dementia. *National Review of Neurology, 7*(6), 323–331.

Carlton, M. (2012, October 13th–14th). Oh for a glimpse of the mum I knew. *Sydney Morning Herald, News Review*, p. 16.

Carnero-Pardo, C. (2014). Should the mini-mental state examination be retired? *Neurologia (English Edition), 29*(8), 473–481.

Chaves, M. L. F. (2014). Cognitive assessment in severe dementia and lower levels of education: Reducing negligence. *Arquivos Neuropsiquiatria, 72*(4), 267–268.

Cheu, S. (2019). Australian ageing agenda. Retrieved August 25, 2020, from https://australianageingagenda.com.au

Coaten, R. (2011). Dance movement therapy in dementia care. In T. Adams, & H. Lee (Eds.), *Creative approaches to dementia care* (pp. 73–90). Palgrave Macmillan.

Dementia Australia. *Tests used in diagnosing dementia.* Dementia Q&A 10. Retrieved June 12, 2022. https://www.dementia.org.au/sites/default/files/helpsheets/Helpsheet-DementiaQandA10-TestsUsedInDiagnosingDementia_english.pdf

Dementia Australia. *Diagnostic criteria for dementia.* Dementia Q&A 11. Retrieved June 12, 2022. https://www.dementia.org.au/sites/default/files/helpsheets/Helpsheet-DementiaQandA11-DiagnosticCriteriaForDementia_english.pdf

Emunah, R. (1994). *Acting for real.* Brunner Mazel, Inc.

Folstein, M., Folstein, S., & McHugh, P. (1975). "Mini-mental state": A practical method for grading the cognitive state of patients for the clinician. *Journal of Psychiatric Resources, 12,* 189–198.

Garrett, K. (2006). Drama therapy can coax Alzheimer's patients back to reality, briefly. *Kansas State University Perspectives, Fall/Winter.* Retrieved November 12, 2019, from https://www.newswise.com/articles/drama-therapy-can-coax-alzheimers-patients-back-to-reality-briefly

Graff-Radford, J. (2020). *Sundowning: Late day confusion.* Retrieved October 20, 2020, from https://www.mayoclinic.org/diseases-conditions/alzheimers-disease/expert-answers/sundowning/faq-20058511

Harrell, L. E., Marson, D., Chatterjee, A., & Parrish, J. A. (2000). The Severe Mini-Mental State Examination: A new neuropsychologic instrument for the bedside assessment of severely impaired patients with Alzheimer disease. *Alzheimer Disease Associative Disorders, 14,* 168–175.

Jaaniste, J. (2011). Dramatherapy and Dementia Care. In H. Lee, & T. Adams (Eds.), *Creative Approaches to Dementia Care* (pp. 54–72). Palgrave Macmillan.

Jaaniste, E. J. (2013). *Pulled through a hedge backwards: Improving the quality of life of people with dementia through dramatherapy* [Unpublished PhD Thesis]. University of Western Sydney.

Kitwood, T. (1997). *Dementia reconsidered.* Open University Press.

Kontos, P., & Martin, W. (2013). Embodiment and dementia: Exploring critical narratives of selfhood, surveillance, and dementia care. *Dementia, 12*(3), 288–302.

Langley, D. (2006). *An introduction to dramatherapy.* Sage Publications.

Lee, H., & Adams, T. (Eds.). (2011). *Creative approaches to dementia care.* Palgrave Macmillan.

McKeith, I., & Cummings, J. (2005). Behavioural changes and psychological symptoms in dementia disorders. *The Lancet (Neurology), 4*(11), 735–742.

Naue, U., & Kroll, T. (2008). The demented other: Identity and difference in dementia. *Nursing Philosophy, 10*(1), 26–33.

Power, G. A. (2011). Foreword. In H. Lee, & T. Adams (Eds.), *Creative approaches in dementia care* (pp. x–xiv). Palgrave MacMillan.

Power, G. A. (2013). *Interview at Dementia Care International.* Retrieved October 10, 2019, from https://dementiacareinternational.com/2013/05/dr-al-power-discusses-spark-of-life-distress-in-dementia/

Power, G. A. (2017). *Dementia beyond disease: Enhancing wellbeing* (Rev. ed.). Health Professions Press, Inc.

Sajnani, N. (2016). *In conversation with Dr Nisha Sajnani.* Retrieved November 27, 2019, from https://blogs.unimelb.edu.au/vcamcm-direct/2016/08/01/in-conversation-with-dr-nisha-sajnani/

Shively, S., Scher, A. I., Perl, D. P., & Diaz-Arrastia, R. (2013). Dementia resulting from traumatic brain injury: What is the pathology? *Archive of Neurology, 69*(10), 1245–1251.

Souter, F. (2015, January 13th). Into the Woods. *Sydney Morning Herald Good Weekend,* pp. 17–19.

Steiner, R. (1985). *On the life of the soul.* Anthroposophic Press.

Steiner, R. (1993). *Understanding the human being* (R. Seddon, Ed.). Rudolf Steiner Press.

Tiwiri, S. C., Tripathi, R. K., & Kumar, A. (2009). Applicability of the mini-mental state examination (MMSE) and the Hindi mental state examination (HMSE) to the urban elderly in India: A pilot study. *International Psychogeriatrics, 21,* 123–128.

Wajeman, J. R., & Bertolucci, P. H. F. (2006). Comparison between neuropsychological evaluation instruments for severe dementia. *Arquivos Neuropsiquiatria, 64,* 736–740.

World Health Organization. (2021). *Dementia fact sheet.* Retrieved June 12, 2022. http://www.who.int/news-room/fact-sheets/detail/dementia

Yaffe, C., Vittinghoff, E., Lindquist, K., Barnes, D., Covinsky, K. E., Kluse, T., & Marmar, M. (2010). Posttraumatic stress disorder and risk of dementia among US veterans. *Archives of General Psychiatry, 67*(6), 608–613.

Yang, H. D., Kim, D. H., & Young, L. D. (2016). History of Alzheimer's disease. *Dementia & Neurocognitive Disorders, 15(4),* 115–121.

Chapter 3

What is dramatherapy?

In the previous chapter, it was suggested that the needs of people with dementia can sometimes be poorly understood. We do know that their signs of distress can often be attributed to assessment according to deficits rather than strengths, disempowering environments, and a lack of genuine human understanding, all adding up to poor quality of life (QoL). There is some evidence that structured, creative engagement in the afternoon would abrogate the need for medication (Graff-Radford, 2020). The arts therapies have much to offer in this area.

Grainger, a dramatherapist who was also an actor and a priest, wrote about the interrelation of dramatherapy and spirituality (Dokter & Carr, 2018). He saw the function of art as being:

> ... always to give form to chaos, definition and identity to a moment or relationship of moments within the flux of events. This is the kind of artistic ability we all possess, and that we use to distinguish among the various functional conventions involving multiple role-playing in a hyper-organised society.
>
> (Grainger, 1995, p. 79)

The body, mind and spirit engagement of this ability is something which persuaded me, during a whole week of afternoon workshops led by Grainger at a summer school in the UK in 1992, to make the decision to become a dramatherapist. As a much younger woman at that time, my understanding was limited, but I now recognise more than a quarter of a century later how important a wholistic approach can be for older people, to allow those with dementia to fully participate in the sorrows and joys of the final life stage.

Like other arts therapies, dramatherapy involves its own drama modality, often including psychotherapy, with the intention of healing. Instead of primarily using visual techniques of art-making, song-making, instrumental music and dance-movement (although sometimes included or applied), dramatherapy uses interventions well-known to theatre. It offers techniques

DOI: 10.4324/9781003186328-3

such as roleplay, improvisation, embodiment and voice work, puppetry and mask-making. There are many methods and techniques of applying drama-therapy (Bailey, 2007). These interventions are offered for the purpose of expressing difficult as well as pleasant emotions and facing significant and sometimes confronting issues in participants' daily lives. In selecting a defi-nition of dramatherapy, Jones (2007) understands local practitioners to offer a more refined sense of the objectives of dramatherapy in a particular context. A local Australian definition is as follows:

> Dramatherapy intentionally uses theatre and drama techniques to encourage the client's creativity and expressive ability.
>
> It helps the clients to tell their story, express feelings, set goals, extend inner experience and try on new and more fulfilling roles, so far unexplored.
>
> Dramatherapy aims to use the imagination to explore ideas, issues and memories and address real-life relationships and social situ-ations through drama. Participants are encouraged to play with their lifescript, telling their story in a new way.
>
> Dramatherapy aims to improve motivation, social skills, self-awareness and self-esteem, developing concepts of responsibility for the self and others in relationships.
>
> (Dramatherapy Centre, 2019)

There is a growing body of qualitative research into the efficacy of drama-therapy with elderly people with mild-to-severe dementia. It is not always possible to have precise information about the diagnoses of dementia, or Alzheimer's disease in particular, and dramatherapists may find themselves working with people whose abilities vary (Langley, 2006, p. 122). When considering the aspects of dramatherapy that are essential applications to engage the elderly, the following can be considered.

Holism – Body, mind and spirit

An especially holistic approach is required for the work of a dramathera-pist, particularly in working with the elderly and those with dementia. The flexibility of dramatherapy with such people comes from the fact that it is based on a fundamental human principle – the way in which we use imag-ination to transform and humanise the world we live in (Anderson-Warren & Grainger, 2000, pp. 18, 22). Dealing first with the physical aspect of the client, one of our core processes of this therapy is embodiment, for example (Jones, 2007). The therapist has an ethical responsibility to the client to be a witness to their body, which may or may not have experienced trauma (Oliver, 2010). In the dramatherapeutic space, the therapist observes the cli-ent, attempting to be as fully aware as possible of what the client wants to communicate, not only verbally but non-verbally as well (Jones, 2007). Jones explains three ways in which dramatherapy's relationship with the client's "dramatic body" can be understood:

> The first area involves clients in developing the potential of their own body. The second area has as its main focus the therapeutic potentials and benefits of the client taking on a different bodily identity within the dramatherapy. The third area concerns work that explores the personal, social and political forces and influences which affect the body.
>
> (Jones, 2007, pp. 228–229)

Embodiment is especially important for physical exercise in this population. The World Health Organization (WHO) recommends that all adults over 65 complete 150 minutes a week of moderate activity such as gardening or walking, or else 75 minutes of more intensive aerobic exercise. This improves cardiac and respiratory health and bone strength, and reduces the risk of falls (WHO, 2020). For people with dementia particularly, even when they have limited physical function, the movement involved in dramatherapy can bring improved physical wellbeing. Regular aerobic and resistance exercise has also proved to be effective in the area of depression among people with dementia (Chen et al., 2017; de Souto Barreto et al., 2015).

Secondly, holism requires a cognitive relationship with the client. Reflection is of paramount importance in this therapy – a reflective intention on the part of the therapist and of the client. Grainger gives this advice:

> A dramatherapist who is trying to find out whether a session of dramatherapy is genuinely therapeutic asks questions about the extent to which a group is succeeding in creating its own shared imaginative 'world'; the degree of awareness that those taking part have of the difference between this and the 'world outside'; the risks that participants are taking in allowing themselves to 'play' in this kind of way and to assume other people's roles; their difficulties in coming back to ordinary reality again.
>
> (Grainger, 1999, p. 116)

In other words, the dramatherapist often needs to elicit from her clients the feeling and thinking behind their experience. The reflection period of any dramatherapy session is extremely significant, when the client can transition from feeling to thinking, assisting them to become more self-aware. Dance movement therapy (DMT) employs rhythm and music to engage clients to reflect in this way. Karkou and Meekums (2017), in their holistic article on DMT with people with dementia, describe "The embodied nature of DMT [which] makes it potentially relevant to those clients for whom body image or body memory may be a particular issue requiring exploration" (2017, pp. 4–5).

People with mild or moderate dementia are still capable of reflection and those with mild dementia of taking on roles. Embodying the role of another can be freeing for that person. De-roling and other distancing techniques which will be more clearly defined later in this book are all helpful in bringing the client back to the here-and-now, so that they may think clearly about what has just taken place dramatically.

Thirdly, the spiritual aspect of the human being needs to be addressed. The word "spirituality" often appears in QoL assessments for people with dementia and others. How do we then define spirituality? For the purposes of this book, my own understanding of spirituality, as opposed to religion, is:

> A holistic and authentic way of being that comes about through awareness of an element or being(s) greater than ourselves and the self weaves certain values into the cloth of a life whose warp and weft include others and nature.
>
> (Jaaniste, 2011, p. 18)

The later chapters of this book are dedicated to significant areas of religion and spirituality, which can be embodied in rituals for mourning and grief or for the celebration of human-to-human sociability.

The warmups used at the beginning of sessions are significant in providing some of the sociability and the movement mentioned above and for releasing any bodily tensions which can reduce flow and flexibility and cause rigidity in the body. As we humans age, our bodies dry up and our limbs and extremities stiffen. This can affect mood, making it easier to isolate and remain immobile. One of the advantages of working in groups is that the participants mirror one another and the collective gives the individual permission to move. There is often a sense of fun and enjoyment – a ball may be thrown around and get missed and it is of no consequence – it usually provokes non-judgmental laughter. Many of the sessions in this book start with games and exercises on a theme, which prepare participants for the main event, which may allow other themes to arise. A collection of images strewn around the floor for people to choose from and play with can act as a warmup also, to help with later projection.

Play

Play comes very naturally to people with dementia, although it has been suggested that in some cases, the willingness to become more creative with frontal lobe deterioration as in dementia can be attributed in some cases to the disinhibition which can accompany the disease (Miller & Miller, 2013). Disinhibition can be difficult for families and carers, as it can be embarrassing when their loved one or client behaves inappropriately in a formal or a social situation. However, in the case of play, it helps them to be more spontaneous than the average adult. Also, unlike clients who have psychosis, people with dementia often appear to have very little resistance to play, whereas psychotic clients are sometimes unwilling to take part in play because it seems childish and they therefore feel infantilised. Disinhibition can also indicate depression and play has many attributes of creative movement and flexibility, which can also be protective factors.

Johnson's (1986) holistic model of dramatherapy known as Developmental Transformations (DvT) gives elderly participants an opportunity to play with end-of-life concerns, while the dramatherapist shifts the scene according to themes which arise during the course of therapy. Smith (2000) shows how the exploration of death anxiety can allay some of the fear and loneliness in people with various levels of dementia, although she states that generally her group members were "relatively cognitively intact". Using case examples, she illustrates the significance of DvT, which allows clients to "confront death anxiety and the existential concerns of freedom and responsibility, isolation and meaninglessness" (pp. 321–322) through imagined scenes of a peaceful afterlife.

The value of play in engaging people with dementia cannot be underrated (Knocker, 2001; Lev-Aladgem, 1999). Lev-Aladgem structures dramatic play using dramatic projection; she uses objects, place and character in a geriatric care centre, in a way that takes dramatherapy further than simply achieving good social and cognitive outcomes. Inspired by Stanislavski's training of actors, she concentrates first on the objects from the clients' environment before moving towards the self. She borrows a walking stick from one of the participants and places it centrally in the circle, whereupon one of the most recognisable symbols of old age is gradually transformed through the imaginations of the participants into a pointer to an imaginary seascape and a hammer which would chop wood. Then she allows the participants to build their own story, culminating in the stick becoming "the post office antelope" (1999, p. 7) whose role is to carry its owner wherever she would like to go. Eventually, she offers the clients a journey from the imaginary world of the projective object to the self. She quotes Courtney (1974) using dramatherapy to "cultivate the 'whole man' and concentrate on the human being's creative imagination" (1999, p. 8).

Lev-Aladgem observes, in common with Gersie (1997), the passive resignation of people waiting out their time in the day centre she visits; obedient, silent and reluctant to make a fuss, until her arrival in the facility and their engagement in active, creative expression (Lev-Aladgem, 1999). In her storytelling with elders, Gersie recognizes that "beneath sullen surface behaviour", these were people who "wanted to surmount these unexamined confines of what old age was supposed to be about" (Gersie, 1997, p. 69). The endless waiting and habitual behaviour are reminiscent of the two tramps in *Waiting for Godot* (Beckett, 2006) as they question their mournful existence while they wait and ask questions. The alternative to the tramps' normal behaviour in the play might be to go on a journey with a client's walking cane, as Lev-Aladgem shows can be possible through "... a stick [which] can provide a stimulus for creative thinking and activity by altering the player's spirit and frame of mind" (1999, p. 7). Another alternative might be to immerse themselves in the world of one of Gersie's (1997) stories of empowerment, where they could find aspects of self they had not recognised before.

Researching dramatherapy

Until recently, little mixed method research has been published concerning dramatherapy groups with participants who are elderly or have dementia and there are few examples of cross-over research involving each of the areas of dementia, dramatherapy and QoL (Jaaniste et al., 2015). An exception to this is the work of Davis Basting's (2006) "Timeslips" story-telling project. Davis Basting uses some dramatherapy and story-making techniques and participants' personal stories are elicited from open-ended questions, the responses to which are creatively developed into narratives. She has been developing theatre techniques for people with dementia for many years (Peters & Katz, 2015), employing imagery and word association to stimulate participants' memories. The Timeslips program research demonstrates improved interpersonal abilities and relationships between staff and clients (Basting, 2006). Johnson (1986) and Sandel and Johnson (1987) use the DvT method to allow the elderly to play, and "to more fully enter the natural flow of time and being, in which each of us is suspended" (Johnson et al., 2003, p. 79). Gorst (2007) shows how, using metaphor, the dramatherapy process can help to redefine the participant's sense of the self-identity that is essential to QoL. The therapy becomes a reflective containment or "two-way street" where the client and therapist use their shared experience of the "timeless moment" as a metaphorical, intersubjective bridge to connect the past, present and future (Gorst, 2007, p. 15). Morris (2011) uses percussive improvisation, character work, games, guided journeys and stories to assist participants to reveal the "unspoken depths" (2011, p. 144) between their creative expression and the "conflicting reality that their brain cells are slowly dying and their futures bleak" (2011, p. 145). She refers, in her existential findings, to the work of Johnson (1991). Dupuis et al. (2016) employ participation in a drama about dementia in a longitudinal arts-based research study to investigate the experiences of living with dementia. They intend to confront stigma in the caring community, and so explore the views on dementia of the family members and carers before and after performing the play entitled I'm still here. The findings showed a profound change in their relationships with the people with dementia in their care.

Collaborative work in the arts therapies

Collaboration between more than one arts therapy can be extremely help-ful for people with dementia. The intergenerational connection between themselves and young people is also encouraging and enlivening for them. A project which calls on both these types of engagement simultaneously is based on the approach of Boal (1979), uniting people with dementia as "spect-actors" with students from a performing arts school (Dassa & Harel, 2019). The combination of music and drama broadens the potential for expression of the participants and singing helps to calm them. The lively support of the young people, who initially show the way by giving a performance of their own, allows greater proactive engagement in the drama. They then include the elderly participants. Because the topic of the musical drama has been drawn from familiar national events in the Israeli environment, and was pre-planned with the potential for improvisation, the people with dementia are able to be reminded of actual biographical experiences in their dramatic expression. They can celebrate personal and collective memories. The engagementgives them agency and a sense of "control, choice as well as dignity" and the inter-generational aspect keeps them grounded (Dassa & Harel, 2019, p. 4).

A dramatherapy session honouring the life stages of people who have mild or moderate Alzheimer's disease

On various occasions, because of my own interest in developmental issues, I have asked groups of all ages to warm up through bodily movement, embod-ying their feelings in their here-and-now life stage. Recognition of cognitive skills has more status in our society than observation of the whole person, such that we can cut off from our body and cease to be in touch with our feelings. Embodiment is the very opposite of disconnection from our physi-cal selves and uses non-verbal movement and symbolic expression (Jennings, 1975; Walsh, 2019). I often ask participants to actively embody themselves at different life stages, moving backwards towards childhood. This exercise is never suggested too early in the life of a group undergoing weekly sessions, as it can be painful and even traumatic until trust has been established. If the group of elders had no dementia, I would begin it in the way described above. I judged that for this group, the method would be too abstract, and so offered embodiment games to warm up and then projection and a gentler form of somatic involvement – walking chronologically from one life stage installa-tion to the next. Thus the projective technique kept the group safe.

For the purposes of this sixth session of 16 with people aged 62–88, in a group consisting of two women and four men, there had been five weekly sessions prior to this one. There had been a group agreement about confi-dentiality and time boundaries, group trust had been established and par-ticipants had gained some idea of what dramatherapy entailed. Through investigation of the results of the Creative Expressive Abilities Assessment (CEAA: Gottlieb-Tanaka et al., 2008), an assessment tool comprising 27 items, which was completed by staff members and art therapy students after each of the group sessions, we were able to monitor the group's progress in seven domains. Staff from the facility and two art therapy students on placement attended the sessions each week and assisted in CEAA observations and recording. We had been able to track the residents' language – verbal as well as non-verbal – as well as evidence of the other six core domains of the tool – memory, attention, sociability, problem-solving, feelings and cultural sharing – as they occurred in the sessions. It was interesting to compare the sessional averages of individuals and groups. We could already discern after five sessions that after an initial weakening in most of these abilities as people got accustomed to being part of the group, there were improvements, especially in the areas of memory, attention, language, problem-solving and emotional expression. This assessment tool is described in greater detail in Chapter 10.

The theme of the session was The joys and woes of memory. The room had been set up before the participants arrived so that they could visit installations corresponding to the developmental phases of their lives. These contained objects related to childhood, adolescence, young adulthood, marriage (they were all married), arrival of children, grandchildren and finally retirement. Some of these projective objects can be seen in Figure 3.1.

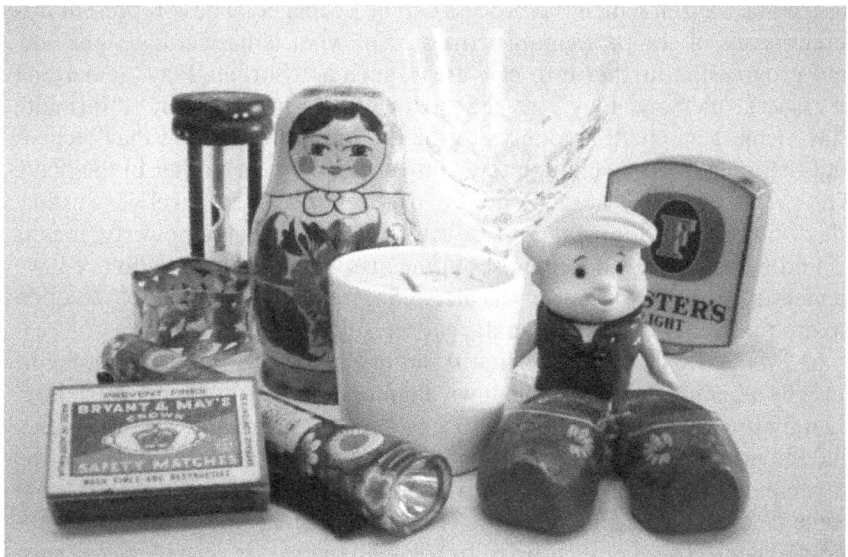

Figure 3.1 Projective objects

Initial discussion and warmups

The session began with conversation about the participants' week. There was a good deal of discussion about Tanya who had experienced a bad fall in the previous week and was not present. Then Ben, a 73-year-old man whose moderate dementia was declining, set the scene in a roundabout way, by describing our activities as "a situation here where everyone's trying to get a hold on something and get going on something and would like and laugh [stet] at doing things. That's the best I am so far that I've come across here". Participants then warmed up with "Shoo, fin, bounce", a game where gestural movement actions around the group were used according to the direction around the circle. The next game was a quick-thinking numbers game, followed by a boisterous sound and movement game, and then they were ready for DvT.

We played "Magic Box", a game from DvT techniques (Johnson, 1986; Sandel & Johnson, 1987). This dramatherapy method had previously proved successful in bringing true feelings to the fore (Jaaniste, 2011), as well as creating a safe space. In DvT group work, the playspace is clearly defined with the participants' help, sharing in the task of making a safe boundary. An important goal of the work is to establish robust intersubjective relationships among participants through clearly defining the environment; encouraging dramatic interaction using voice and embodiment; allowing meaningful integration through reminiscence and re-membering improvisation, and being unafraid to refer to bodily limitations and end-of-life issues (Johnson, 1986; Johnson et al., 1982). Johnson (2009) recommends a series of ways in which the process can be deepened. These represent different levels of the participant letting go of what is happening right now and progressing further into new areas, such as "Surface Play" (emerging of issues); "Persona Play" (re-enactment of significant others); "Intimate Play" (emergent client responses to the therapist), and "Deep Play" (client and therapist freed up enough to be unrestricted by each other in the play). The clients described here did not go any deeper than the level of "Surface Play"; however, as Johnson reports, this level of playing is a powerful means of finding new roles and being spontaneous. With clients who do not have dementia, all of the deeper levels after "Surface Play" are possible to open up gradually and fuel the dramatic action (Johnson, 2009, p. 95).

In "Magic Box", the clients first stand in a circle and the therapist facilitates by assisting them to bring down an imaginary curtain from the ceiling, then finding a gap in the curtain to step through, engaging with the scene, and moving it along according to what she observes and understands of the participants. It is then part of her role as facilitator to anticipate potential scene changes according to an awareness of themes and group and individual needs. The therapist helps to "define" themes or activities, and then "identifying", asking participants what it reminds them of, until they are ready for a "personification" or role-playing stage (Johnson, 1986; Johnson et al., 1982). The therapist needs to enter the improvisation in order to move the action along. At all times, there should be an awareness of themes, and what kinds of themes are emerging, often from their personal material. For people with dementia, the therapist needs to take an active role, repeating and reiterating the clients' comments in line with emerging themes and asking questions such as "Who are you now?" or "Are you still the treasure-seeker?" in order to stay with or advance the role-play.

After several interactions which included a flying cockroach and the discovery of an old treasure box hiding gold, the theme of memory came up, assisted by the metaphor of the hidden treasure. Leanne, a 70-year-old woman with mild dementia, said that she had been emotionally abused by a teacher who prevented her from playing during the breaks at primary school, and never explained why. The experience was a betrayal by the teacher which had taught her to hate.

As suggested by Johnson, the "Magic Box" can later become an "Emotional Soup" (Johnson, 1986, p. 23). Participants can pull out emotions and return them to the soup with sounds and facial expressions. This was a painful memory from childhood that Leanne had reportedly been obsessed with, reiterating it at home and in other group sessions at the day centre. I had already tried, unsuccessfully, to open up this memory through roleplay. Still in the playspace, and inspired by Leanne's contribution, participants were asked to throw unpleasant memories into a cauldron. Each participant responded in turn with an unwanted memory, and then was asked where they would like to put the vessel with its "murky contents". They chose to put it outside, so we managed to bring it out from the curtained play space, making sure we returned the curtain to the ceiling, and took the imaginary cauldron outside the French doors and into the garden.[1]

With the cauldron safely outside, participants were invited to the various life stage installations of the room, described earlier. Responses to these visitations were as follows: in the section entitled "childhood", we found out that Neil (62, with mild dementia) had a favourite memory of being read to in bed at nights by parents, and this is where his love of stories came from. David (74 years old with unspecified dementia) told us about his dog: "With Juna with you - beside us, no one sort of interfered with us seeing we had a dog like that. It was a beautiful dog". The animal was extremely important to this man, since he had been at a boarding school in New South Wales with an outrageous history of child abuse. He never disclosed actual abuse, but certainly improvised and role-played himself in a later session hiding from the Catholic Brothers while at school (see Chapter 7). Juna also turned up again in the program. We learned that Leanne had loved the freedom of roller skates, and Ben (73, with moderate Alzheimer's) was glad he wasn't good at football because "They have to a) be seen; b) get hold of them and c) make sure you do because you've got to use them".

Moving on to the next stage, Neil freely told us about the problems of his adolescence: "And, ah, but it – but there's sort of a, what do you say, wasn't all smooth. Yeah. A difficult time but it was also a growing time, you know. And you have to grow through it otherwise you died". Paul (88, with Parkinson's related dementia) said he was introduced to girls and went dancing. Leanne sadly told us that she didn't go out, but stayed home to make her own clothes: "Cause my mum and dad were not very wealthy … They got better later but at that time it was hand to mouth almost, you know".

These life stage themes were foundational and revealed a great deal about the participants and their ups and downs in their formative years. In the absence of a genogram, it was a great way to start to understand a little about the earlier years of participants. As Landau (2018, p. 69) writes in his article on meaning and metaphor: "Among the many strategies for finding meaning in life, metaphor use is remarkable because it involves an ability, unique to humans, to comprehend how two concepts share a similar structure despite their superficial differences". In other words, for Leanne, the narrative of her childhood and adolescent life told us so much about the importance of her ability to play.

The group walked on to the "working life" area after leaving school. Once more, we found that Ben's story was more about what he was not able or allowed to do – he lived near the big grammar school, but was not involved with it. He lived in that area, but had no money so "had to walk". Paul said: "… there was a sort of degree of, ah, being able to think about what you were doing and do it because you wanted to do it, and such like things. Reading. Able to study books". Leanne went on to become a teacher, and a very different teacher from the woman who had emotionally abused her, who "just did not play the game right". David became a solicitor through the Solicitors Admission Board, and Neil said:

> I didn't become an adult until I was around about 30. I suppose it was delayed because of, um, university and a lot of training and, um, stuff like that. So, um, yeah, that just came to me, that adulthood really was held back a bit because of all those studies.

The participants moved on to the marriage section – I called it that because all of them had been or were presently married. In all cases, it was their partner who brought them to the sessions every week. Neil said: "J – is my lover, full stop". Paul had only ever wanted one wife. Ben said: "it's been an extraordinarily good way to go and that occurs for me and my wife which is good and, um, we have five or so kids". Leanne said of marriage: "I like it. And my husband is a very nice man. A beautiful man". David said it was a great institution and he had been married twice and had five children. This was the cue to move to the next stopping place – the "birth of children" corner.

Passing through the children and grandchildrens' corners, the participants were invited to go back the way they had come through the life stages, taking objects from anywhere they wished. It was interesting to see how they experienced life stages through projection.

David picked up an egg timer from the "grandparent" section, which showed him the sands of time would run out for him, as for others. He expressed the reality of the approach of death and the end that comes to all humans in their later life stages. Leanne picked up a baby photo from the "childhood" section, and said, "I love children". It was poignant after her toxic memory earlier in the session that she took the photo of the innocent child, rather than the one who had been taught to hate.

In the "working life" section, Neil picked up a picture of a soldier. For him, this represented his father, who had fought in World War Two. He told us the picture "reminded me that, um, that my father has died, um, but, ah, and there's something about his dying that left me with, um, some grief or unresolved matter".

Then Neil had the realisation that there was unfinished business for him connected with the death of his father, showing the importance of projection for him and for the participants generally. By walking through once and experiencing memories through the embodiment within a particular life stage area, the strong sense of connection that was experienced on the way back when he could choose an object gave it more meaning. Neil had opened up a memory which he was able to work with in a further session, which will be related in Chapter 8. Dramatherapy shows ways in which dramatic projection can be associated with other dramatic forms to help clients "create, discover and engage with external representations of inner conflicts" (Jones, 2007, p. 140). Armstrong et al. (2016) found in their quantitative research that dramatic embodiment and dramatic projection are both observable, as indeed they were in this instance.

In the following chapter, there will be more focus on the QoL of elders and people with dementia and how dramatherapy can improve resilience and well-being for people later in the lifespan.

Note

1 There will be more later in the book about Leanne's story, and it is interesting that it came up so early in this session. This early stage of Leanne's work with childhood trauma will be re-visited in Chapter 7: Trauma and intersubjectivity in dementia.

References

Anderson-Warren, M., & Grainger., R. (2000). *Practical approaches to dramatherapy.* Jessica Kingsley.

Armstrong, C. R., Rozenberg, M., Powell, M. A., Honce, J., Honstein, L., Gingras, G., & Han, E. (2016). A step toward empirical operationalizing and uncovering dramatherapy change processes. *The Arts in Psychotherapy*, *49*, 27–33.

Bailey, S. (2007). Drama therapy. In A. Blatner (Ed.), *Interactive improvisational drama* (pp. 164–173). iUniverse.

Beckett, S. (2006). *Waiting for Godot*. Faber & Faber.

Boal, A. (1979). *Theatre of the oppressed*. Pluto Press.

Chen, K.-M., Huo, C.-C., Chang, Y.-H., Huang, H.-T., & Cheng, Y.-Y. (2017). Resistance band exercises reduce depression and behavioural problems of wheelchair-bound older adults with dementia: A cluster randomized control trial. *Journal of the American Geriatric Society*, *65*(2), 356–363.

Dassa, A., & Harel, D. (2019). People with dementia as "spect-actors" in a musical theatre group with performing arts students from the community. *The Arts in Psychotherapy*, *65*(101592), 1–6.

Basting, D. (2006). Arts in dementia care: This is not the end ... it's the end of this chapter. *Generations*, *30*(1), 16–20.

de Souto Barreto, P., Demougeot, L., Pillard, F., Lapeyre-Meistre, M., & Yves, R. (2015). Exercise training for managing behavioural and psychological symptoms in people with dementia: A systematic review and meta-analysis. *Ageing Research Reviews*, *24*, 274–285.

Dokter, D., & Carr, M. (2018). Drama and religion: (Un)comfortable bedfellows? In honour of Dr. Roger Grainger. *Dramatherapy*, *39*(1), 16–28.

Dramatherapy Centre. Retrieved October 10, 2019, from www.dramatherapy.com.au

Dupuis, S. L., Mitchell, G. J., Jonas-Simpson, C. M., Whyte, C. P., Gillies, J. L., & Carson, J. D. (2016). Igniting transformative change in dementia care through research-based drama. *The Gerontologist*, *56*(6), 979–989.

Gersie, A. (1997). *Reflections on therapeutic storymaking*. Jessica Kingsley.

Gorst, A. (2007). Awakening from the dream of thought: Research into dramatherapy and dementia. *Dramatherapy*, *29*(2), 10–16.

Gottlieb-Tanaka, D., Lee, H., & Graf, P. (2008). *Creative-expressive abilities assessment: User guide*. ArtScience Press.

Graff-Radford, J. (2020). Sundowning: late day confusion. Retrieved October 20, 2020, from https://www.mayoclinic.org/diseases-conditions/alzheimers-disease/expert-answers/sundowning/faq-20058511

Grainger, R. (1995). *The glass of heaven: The faith of the dramatherapist*. Jessica Kingsley.

Grainger, R. (1999). *Researching the arts therapies: A dramatherapist's perspective*. Jessica Kingsley.

Jaaniste, J. (2011). Dramatherapy and spirituality in dementia care. *Dramatherapy*, *33*(1), 16–27.

Jaaniste, J., Linnell, S., Ollerton, R. L., & Slewa-Younan, S. (2015). Dramatherapy with older people with dementia: Does it improve quality of life? *Arts in Psychotherapy*, *43*, 40–48.

Jennings, S. (1975). The importance of the body in non-verbal methods of therapy. In S. Jennings (Ed.), *Creative therapy*. Pitman.

Johnson, D. (1986). The developmental method in dramatherapy: Group treatment with the elderly. *The Arts in Psychotherapy*, *13*, 17–33.

Johnson, D. (1991). The theory and technique of transformations in drama therapy. *The Arts in Psychotherapy*, *18*(4), 285–300.

Johnson, D. (2009). Developmental transformations: Towards the body as a presence. In D. Johnson & R. Emunah (Eds.), *Current approaches in dramatherapy* (2nd ed., pp. 89–116). Charles C. Thomas.

Johnson, D., Sandel, S., & Margolis, M. (1982). Principles of group treatment in a nursing home. *Journal of Long-Term Care Administration*, *10*, 19–24.

Johnson, D., Smith, A., & James, M. (2003). Developmental transformations in group therapy with the elderly. In C. E. Schaefer (Ed.), *Play therapy with adults* (pp. 78–103). John Wiley & Sons.

Jones, P. (2007). *Drama as therapy: Theory, practice and research* (2nd ed.). Routledge.

Karkou, V., & Meekums, B. (2017). Dance movement therapy for dementia. *Cochrane Database of Systematic Reviews*, *2*, 1–24.

Knocker, S. (2001). A meeting of worlds: Play and metaphor in dementia care and dramatherapy. *Dramatherapy*, *23*(2), 4–9.

Landau, M. J. (2018). Using metaphor to find meaning in life. *Review of General Psychology American Psychological Association*, *22*(1), 62–72.

Langley, D. (2006). *An introduction to dramatherapy*. Sage Publications.

Lev-Aladgem, S. (1999). Dramatic play amongst the aged. *Dramatherapy*, *21*(3), 3–10.

Miller, Z. A., & Miller, B. L. (2013). Artistic creativity and dementia. *Progress in Brain Research*, *21*(204), 99–112.

Morris, N. (2011). Unspoken depths: Dramatherapy and dementia. *Dramatherapy*, *33*(3), 144–157.

Oliver, S. A. (2010). Trauma, bodies and performance art: Towards an embodied ethics of seeing. *Continuum*, *24*(1), 119–129.

Peters, R., & Katz, S. (2015). Interview with Dr Anne Davis Basting, 21 May 2013. *Dementia*, *14*(3), 328–334.

Sandel, S., & Johnson, D. (1987). *Waiting at the gate: Creativity & hope in the nursing home*. The Haworth Press.

Smith, A. (2000). Exploring the death anxiety with older adults through developmental transformations. *Arts in Psychotherapy*, *27*, 321–332.

Walsh, M., *Embodied facilitator*. Retrieved December 18, 2019, from https://embodiedfacilitator.com/

World Health Organization. (2020). Physical activity and older adults. Retrieved August 24, 2020, from https://www.who.int/dietphysicalactivity/factsheet_olderadults/en/

Chapter 4

Dramatherapy, dementia and quality of life: A research project

A review of the literature deals with other arts therapies and dramatherapy approaches supporting people who have dementia. A description of a dramatherapy session with people who have dementia, visiting installations of the various lifestages they have been through, is presented as an example of how this modality can support them in honouring their lives so far. Readers are offered insights into participants' lives as they move from one remembered stage of development to another, encouraged to picture the trajectory of their lives as a whole. Developmental connections and reminiscence give readers an informed sense of sessional outcomes.

I had believed for some time before starting the research project described in this chapter that dramatherapy may improve the behavioural and psychological symptoms of dementia (BPSD), but also participants' quality of life (QoL). As I wrote some years later in 2021, there is more discourse about what can affect QoL: for example, co-morbidity with other conditions (Nelis et al., 2019), structural characteristics of the environment (Palm et al., 2019), and relationships (O'Rourke et al., 2015). At the current Royal Commission into Aged Care, the word "life" is not paired with "quality" in their theme of Quality and Safety. The discourse is more about risk management. Their rubric is to some extent understandable, since there has been so much publicity about the abuse of people in care homes; however, I believe the word "life" should still stand, associated with quality. My concern includes research on the inappropriate and habituated use of anti-psychotic medication (Almutairi et al., 2018; Phillips, 2016). This systematic offering of such medication by care staff described by these thinkers may have some influence on the fact that the launch of the English national dementia strategy did not result in a reduction of anti-psychotic prescribing in care homes at all after four years (Szczepura et al., 2016). It is worthwhile to explore the ways QoL has been seen and measured in the recent past, for the purposes of connecting it with suitable dramatherapy interventions.

DOI: 10.4324/9781003186328-4

Quality of life and dementia

QoL is a complex area because of the inherent problems in defining this term and the fact that it invariably means different things to different people. Older adults consistently indicate that well-being and QoL are more relevant than disease-related outcomes and it can be ascertained with accuracy in people with dementia (Hoe et al., 2007). Encompassing the treatment of the whole person, QoL has been defined in various ways. Phenomena encountered in this research project spoke volumes about the following qualities described in a survey of people with dementia who lived in the community and were asked, sometimes with the help of picture cards and talking mats, what they believed were the most important features of QoL. Some of these were the attributes of family, physical health, independence, relationships, communication and "who I am" (Alzheimer's Society, 2010).

There is a general consensus that QoL typically includes physical, psychological, social and emotional areas of well-being and resilience (Birren & Diekermann, 1991; Moyle et al., 2007). Resilience is about overcoming obstacles, being flexible, and not necessarily springing back into the same habits after adverse circumstances, but finding a new way of being. Moyle, with other authors, views QoL in dementia as having been largely ignored and worthy of much greater examination (Moyle et al., 2007). These authors have a strong belief in client choice and agency where at all possible, pointing out that an assessment of QoL should incorporate the perspective of the person with dementia. They compared two reliable and widely used assessment tools which encouraged this process: Quality of Life Alzheimer's disease (QoL-AD) (Logsden et al., 1999) and the Dementia Quality of Life Questionnaire (DQL). (The QoL-AD was also the scale chosen for my study below.) From a group of 61 people with dementia in long-term care, 60 filled out the former and 40 the latter questionnaires. Although both scales were able to elicit the participants' perspective on QoL, the QoL-AD was more user-friendly. In 2011, the authors (Moyle et al., 2011) went on to use the QoL-AD only with people with dementia, triangulated with proxies: a carer and a family member in each case. They found that the people with dementia gave themselves higher ratings than their proxies did. This was partly because the proxies' assessments were associated with activities of daily living (ADLs) with reduced QoL consideration connected with limitations on activity (Moyle et al., 2011).

Wendy Moyle is an adherent of the person-centred paradigm which influences many of the arguments in my study below. Connected with this paradigm, Brod et al. (1999) indicated that the person's own appraisal (rather than relying on objective observations) of their personal and environmental circumstances leads to the QoL experienced by the individual. Person-centred care demands the centrality of subjective measures for the elderly (Merchant & Hope, 2004).

Person-centred care

Person-centred care is a much more holistic alternative to conventional care practices (Brooker, 2004; Loveday et al., 1998). This type of care replaces the effects of malignant social psychology (Kitwood, 1997), keeping the client at the centre of their world rather than othering them. Care that is holistic can soften the blow where there is cognitive and functional deterioration (Chenoweth et al., 2009). Kitwood and Bredin (1992) saw the relationship of the person with dementia as being one of communication with others, where signs of well-being were such aspects as initiating social connection, using humour and creative self-expression, which indicate that their personhood remains intact even though they have dementia (Knocker, 2001). The practice of person-centred care in facilities for people with dementia that prioritises their individual interests, background and needs leads to dignity, independence and better QoL for such people. It often requires staff training in active listening and learning, but once it is established, it can free them and their staff from agitation, anxiety and stress (Careabout Advisory Service, 2019).

Quality of life and spirituality

In a report by the UK-based Alzheimer's Society (2010), people with dementia were asked to identify their most important elements of QoL. With the help of flashcards and talking mats, they worked out their priorities, one of which was freedom to practise faith or religion. Among the 44 participants in the research, all of whom had mild to severe dementia, 16 were from black and minority ethnic groups. It is of great importance to pay attention to diversity and give people the opportunity to talk about their faith or religion. Towako Katsumo (2005, pp. 332–333) specifically addresses spirituality and remarks that healthcare professionals should try to fulfil three main requirements:

- To understand and respect a person's spiritual beliefs
- To provide spiritual care for people with dementing illnesses in educational programmes
- To include standardised questionnaires for assessing the personal spirituality of people with dementia

All three of these conditions are or can be met by a dramatherapist. Personally, I believe QoL which includes spiritual care and a respect for any religious beliefs of people with dementia can be termed "experiential well-being", which is at the heart of my thesis. Krieger and Hanson (1999) argue for the importance of the spiritual element, suggesting that one meaning of "to be healthy" is "to be whole", and to experience wholeness is the very essence of what it is to be spiritual (Krieger & Hanson, 1999, p. 305). Margaret Goodall (2009, p. 167) believes that "all good care should have a strong spiritual dimension at its heart", and Shamy believes that although it is far more difficult for a carer to neglect a person's physical difficulties than their spiritual needs, it is essential that their non-corporeal rights be observed as well (Shamy, 1997).

Pulled through a hedge backwards: Can dramatherapy improve the quality of life of people with dementia?

In a PhD research project testing this hypothesis, a mixed method approach was chosen where I wore two hats: that of the therapist and that of the researcher (Jaaniste, 2013). Having worked in a few aged care centres, I was not convinced that people with dementia were being offered the kinds of therapies which would call upon their creativity to help them find meaning in their day-to-day lives.

Method

Under the rubric of an Australian organisation providing daycare centres for people with dementia, a two-arm study was set up with a group of nine participants enrolled in movie-watching sessions in their Newcastle, NSW facility, while a group of six undertook dramatherapy sessions in their Sydney centre. Participants in the fieldwork all lived in the community and had been given mixed diagnoses by their medical practitioners, although most were diagnosed with Alzheimer's disease (AD). Both groups ran for 16 sessions, with a midway break of three weeks. Participants in both groups were assessed using a neuropsychological test pre- and post-groupwork for QoL (as seen in Figure 4.1). All six members of the dramatherapy group were qualitatively evaluated using phenomenological epistemology, ethnography, narrative and metaphor analysis.

Ethics

For this study, approved by the Ethics Committee of Western Sydney University, release forms were discussed with and signed by participants and their carers, to give permission for the research to be published. No permission was given to show images of the volunteers.

> It is an ethical priority in the care of people with dementia to maximise the likelihood that they will have opportunities to live lives reflective of their values and maintain active, central roles in decision-making.
>
> (Wilkins, 2017, p. 637)

Clearly, decisions such as these should be made on a case-by-case basis and valid consent must be sought. Carers need to be involved in such decisions,

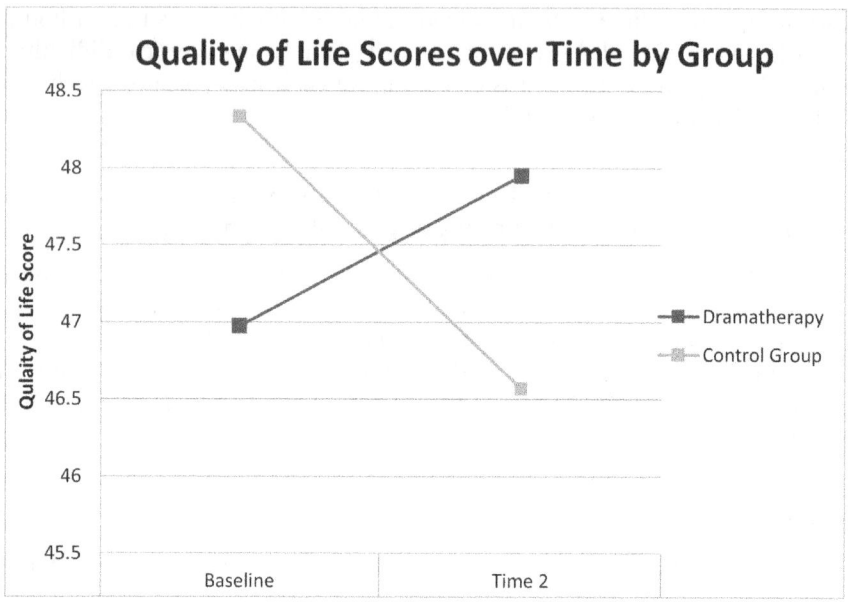

Figure 4.1 Quality of life scores over time

but as the American Art Therapy Association (2020) advises in their section on autonomy for clients, where possible their views should be respected in their decision-making throughout the process. With regard to the ethics of research, Sarah Anacleto (2018) reports a situation where a client has painted a dynamic picture, yet was discontented with the result and could barely approach it. Although, as the researcher, she had previously been given officially signed consent to photograph it, the client changed her mind, and she wished it to be disposed of. In order to truly respect the client's autonomy, Sarah had to face the uncomfortable challenge that her wish to have a full portfolio of her work as a research subject was now impossible. Once she realised this, she was able to respect and validate the client's request to destroy the painting. In other words, Sarah declined to reinforce the stigma of dementia that sadly exists among some members of the community.

Why choose a mixed method approach?

Analysis on both sides of the methodological – qualitative/quantitative – divide is very significant in my own working life, as so much of the previous 15 years before writing up the research had been as a dramatherapist working in the mental health area. In our Australian mental health system, the biomedical model often looks for a standardised form of evidence-based practice (EBP) which quantitative research can provide. The search for EBP in dementia has in the past provided pathways to the goal of accurately diagnosing the condition before death. As mentioned above, not long ago, people had to die before having their brains autopsied to show beyond any doubt that amyloid plaque and other brain changes cause dementia. This process ensured a more exact post-mortem diagnosis, or detected a misdiagnosis (Kolata, 2010). Later research has led to the discovery of shrinkage in the brain through MRI scans and uptake of glucose to show brain activity through PET scans (Johnson et al., 2012). These innovations have been reached through rigorous research culminating in EBP for diagnosing dementia.

Quantitative research and its ability to identify patterns in the data is regarded as best practice in the biomedical domain. Even though there is evidence, now provided by quantum physicists, that such patterns may be subjectively influenced and therefore, scientifically unreliable (Schwarz & Begley, 2003), deduction in research from quantitative data is the preferred method of capturing information for best practice. Having spent many years working in this domain, I wanted to be able to show in a modest way, yet justifiably, that dramatherapists are able to speak the language of physicists, despite difficulties associated with quantifying the arts therapies.

"Dramatherapy ... sometimes appears to shy away from both things - interpretation and measurement!" (Grainger, 1999, p. 15). However, Caul and Gaugler (2014) have shown in their systematic review of the efficacy of Creative Arts Therapies (CATs) in the treatment of AD and dementia that statistical significance was achieved for most of the randomised controlled trials studied despite small sample sizes (ranging from 18 to 60). These results provide quantitative evidence for the beneficial role of creative arts. However, Grainger's views are substantiated even here, because out of 63 quantitative or mixed method articles there were only two offering dramatherapy alone, and none investigating via randomised control trials (RCTs). One study was by Fritsch et al. (2006), who found improvements in engagement and affect of their participants, as well as staff involved having improved interaction with residents, job satisfaction, attitude towards residents and decreased rates of burnout. The other was a study by Wilkinson et al. (1998), who found improvement in cognition, mood, ADLs and depression.

A collaborative article (Jaaniste et al., 2015) was published later than Caul and Gaugler's (2014) review, where our investigation had numbers at the smaller end (13); however, when the quantitative QoL data were triangulated with the qualitative results, "an unambiguous participant ability to express ideas and feelings through dramatherapy" (Jaaniste et al., 2015, p. 40) emerged. In addition, there was, "an unveiling of conscious awareness of participants' own wellbeing and QoL" (2015, p. 40). The findings also indicate that a future larger study needs to be undertaken along similar lines to those in our study.

Quantitative and qualitative approaches possess differing characteristics for practice. Grainger (1999) quotes Maxwell (1996, p. 9): "Quantitative approaches are powerful ways of determining whether a particular result was causally related to one or another variable, and to what extent these are related". He continues by pointing out that qualitative research is often better at demonstrating "how" the change happened. In other words, for those who are interested in the amount of change dramatherapy produces by way of outcomes, in their own positivist terms, quantitative approaches are best. For those who want to know "how" these outcomes are produced so that aims for healing can be achieved more cogently, qualitative assessment works best (Grainger, 1999).

This dual role of a mixed method investigation demonstrates to the sceptical within the biomedical system that deductive quantitative research does not present the whole picture. In this book, I hope the "how" of the research can be found in the phenomenological evidence within its pages. The acts and voices of the participants as well as the intersubjectivity of the dramatherapist and group members are there to demonstrate what can occur in varied areas of practice. The qualitative areas – the metaphorical, ethnographic and narrative used in the project – are positioned to lift the veil from the invisibility of people with dementia. These methods of analysis aim to demonstrate the existence of conscious wisdom in elders, despite (and perhaps because of!) their disabilities. Qualitative enquiry "knows how" to do this, whereas quantitative research displays a certain rigour in juggling with variables that may be absent from the former method. Rigour is also needed in vigorous qualitative enquiry of course; however, this qualitative order of rigour may not always be recognised by scientifically trained people who are unaware of phenomenological ontology or do not take it seriously (Jaaniste, 2013).

Investigation results

Two members of the dramatherapy group experienced serious falls outside of sessions and were hospitalised and unable to continue. The QoL-AD (Logsdon et al., 1999), a 13-item self-assessment and caregiver measure of QoL, was used for the assessment. The data produced by the participants were weighted more heavily in the analysis than their carers', in answer to the same questions. The samples were not statistically significant in age $t(11) = 0.797$, $p = 0.46$ or gender, $\chi^2(1, n = 13) = 2.44$, $p = 0.308$. When examining the levels of educational attainment between the two groups, no significant difference was noted, $\chi^2(1, n = 13) = 1.935$, $p = 0.27$. Finally, no differences between the types of dementia were noted between the two groups $\chi^2(1, n = 13) = 2.438$, $p = 0.308$.

Although not statistically significant, the dramatherapy group's scores increased on average by 1.0 (rounded) from T1 and the Film Group's decreased on average by 1.8 (rounded) from T1 QoL-AD; T2–T1; p = 0.33 as seen in Figure 4.1. The QoL-AD was demonstrated to have been the right scale to use to assess all 13 completing participants from the two groups.

The quantitative difference in scores may be attributed to low numbers in the study, or it may be circumspect to assume that there was an improvement in QoL. The research was triangulated with the observation and in-depth analysis of the sessions, and I was able to ascertain that dramatherapy is a promising treatment for enhancing the QoL of people living with dementia. Names were changed for the purposes of publication and releases signed by participants.

Discussion

The mixed method enquiry established QoL as a robust and essential element of existence which can emerge from the person-centred respect that we owe to elders with dementia. Additionally, a recognition and valuing of their holistic physical, spiritual, social and psychological needs are significant constituent aspects of QoL. The study aimed to challenge the dominant view that the life led by many elders is no longer fully human and that medication is essential. The study broadened the debate about dementia in the community, showing that a more empathic approach, giving agency where possible to the person with dementia, is a realistic aim. This can occur without a primary reliance on anti-psychotic medication for restlessness and aggression. The qualitative arm of the research has also shown that people with mild, moderate or even early severe dementia have a high level of self-awareness which can be engaged and this is not apparent from the biomedical literature (Jaaniste, 2014). In addition, this study has broadened the debate on the use of mixed methods in this type of research. To my knowledge, there has been no other ethically approved mixed methods study using dramatherapy on the QoL of people with dementia.

Conclusion

Qualitatively, the research revealed a surprising ability of the participants to self-heal, to self-advocate and to have a voice in the world. They also exhibited a conscious appreciation of their situation which I had not expected. They expressed difficult feelings without in any way showing restlessness or aggression attributable to BPSD; on the contrary, they were socially engaged in this process, as can be observed from the discussion of phenomenological observations below. These aspects of the research are considered in relation to the themes of independence, relationships, communication and "who I am" – three of the aspects of QoL chosen by the cohort of participants in the Alzheimer's Society (2010) research mentioned above. They also showed a sense of empathy towards self, sometimes including others, which will be explained in the following chapter.

References

Almutairi, S., Masters, K., & Donyai, P. (2018). The health professional experience of using antipsychotic medication for dementia in care homes: A study using grounded theory and focussing on inappropriate prescribing. *Journal of Psychiatric Mental Health Nursing*, *25*, 307–318.

Alzheimer's Society. (2010). *My name is not dementia: People with dementia discuss quality of life indicators*. Author. https://www.yumpu.com/en/document/view/32296908/alzheimers-society-my-name-is-not-dementia-people-with

American Art Therapy Association. (2020). Aspirational values underlying the ethical principles for art therapists. https://arttherapy.org/wp-content/uploads/2017/06/Aspirational-Values-Underlying-the-Ethical-Principles-for-Art-Therapists.pdf

Anacleto, S. (2018). Aspirational ethics: Considerations for art therapy practice in a health care setting for adults with dementia. *Journal of the American Art Therapy Association*, *35*(3), 165–169.

Birren, J., & Diekermann, L. (1991). Concepts and content of quality of life in later years: An overview. In J. Birren, J. Lubben, & J. C. Rowe (Eds.), *Concept and measurement of quality of life in the frail elderly* (pp. 344–360). Academic Press.

Brod, M., Stewart, A. L., Sands, L., & Walton, P. (1999). Conceptualisation of quality of life in dementia: The quality of life instrument (DQoL). *The Gerontologist*, *39*(1), 25–35.

Brooker, D. (2004). What is person-centred care in dementia? *Review of Clinical Gerontology*, *13*, 215–222.

Careabout Advisory Service. (2019). *Person centred dementia care*. Retrieved on February 20, 2020, from https://www.careabout.com.au/blog/person-centered-dementia-care

Caul, A. L., & Gaugler, J. L. (2014). Efficacy of creative arts therapy in treatment of Alzheimer's disease and dementia: A systematic review. *Activities Adaptation & Aging*, *38*(4), 281–330.

Chenoweth, L., King, M. T., Jeon, Y.-H., Brodaty, H., Stein-Parbury, J., Norman, R., Haas, M., & Luscombe, G. (2009). Caring for aged dementia care resident study (CADRES) of person-centred care, dementia care mapping and usual care in dementia: A cluster-randomised trial. *The Lancet Neurology*, *8*(4), 317–325.

Fritsch, T., Betts Adams, K., Redd, D., Sias, T., & Herrup, K. (2006). Use of live theater to increase minority participation in Alzheimer disease research. *Alzheimer Disease and Associated Disorders*, *20*(2), 105–111.

Goodall, M. (2009). The evaluation of spiritual care in a dementia care setting. *Dementia*, *8*(2), 167–183.

Grainger, R. (1999). *Researching the arts therapies: A dramatherapist's perspective*. Jessica Kingsley.

Hoe, J., Katona, C., Orrell, M., & Livingston, G. (2007). Quality of life in dementia: Care recipient and caregiver perceptions of quality of life in dementia: The LASER-AD study. *International Journal of Geriatric Psychiatry*, *22*, 1031–1036.

Jaaniste, E. J. (2013). *Pulled through a hedge backwards: Improving the quality of life of people with dementia through dramatherapy* [Unpublished PhD Thesis]. University of Western Sydney.

Jaaniste, J. (2014). Missing the point: Dementia, biomedicine & dramatherapy. In I. Veljanova, C. Mills, & G. Emmanuel (Eds.), *Health, agency and wellbeing* (pp. 3–16). Inter-Disciplinary Press.

Jaaniste, J., Linnell, S., Ollerton, R. L., & Slewa-Younan, S. (2015). Dramatherapy with older people with dementia: Does it improve quality of life? *Arts in Psychotherapy, 43*, 40–48.

Johnson, K. A., Fox, N. C., Sperling, R. A., & Klunk, W. E. (2012). Brain imaging in Alzheimer disease. *Cold Spring Harbor Perspectives in Medicine, 2*(4), a006213.

Katsumo, T. (2005). Dementia from the inside: How people with early-stage dementia evaluate their quality of life. *Ageing and Society, 25*(2), 197–214.

Kitwood, T. (1997). *Dementia reconsidered.* Open University Press.

Kitwood, T., & Bredin, K. (1992). Towards a theory of dementia care: Personhood and wellbeing. *Ageing & Society, 12*(3), 269–287.

Knocker, S. (2001). A meeting of worlds: Play and metaphor in dementia care and dramatherapy. *Dramatherapy, vol. 23*(2), 4–9.

Kolata, G. (2010, June 24). Test may open door to spotting Alzheimer's. *International Herald Tribune, 23*, pp. 1, 8.

Krieger, M. P., & Hanson, B. J. (1999). A value-based paradigm for creating truly healthy organisations. *Journal of Organisational Change Management, 12*(4), 302–317.

Logsdon, R., Gibbons, L., McCurry, S., & Teri, L. (1999). Quality of life in Alzheimer's disease: Patient and caregiver reports. *Journal of Mental Health & Ageing, 5*, 21–32.

Loveday, B., Kitwood, T., & Bowe, B. (1998). *Improving dementia care.* Hawker Publications Ltd.

Maxwell, J. A. (1996). *Qualitative research design: An interactive approach.* Sage Publications.

Merchant, C., & Hope, K. (2004). The quality of life in Alzheimer's disease scale: Direct assessment of people with cognitive impairment. *International Journal of Older People Nursing in association with Journal of Clinical Nursing, 13*(6b), 105–110.

Moyle, W., McAllister, M., Venturato, L., & Adams, T. (2007). Quality of life & dementia. *Dementia, 6*(2), 175–191.

Moyle, W., Murfield, J. E., Griffiths, S. G., & Venturato, L. (2011). Assessing quality of life of older people with dementia: A comparison of quantitative self-report and proxy accounts. *Journal of Advanced Nursing, 68*(10), 2237–2246.

Nelis, S. M., Wu, Y. T., Matthews, F. E., Martyr, A., Quinn, C., Rippon, I., Rusted, J., Thom, J. M., Kopelman, M. D., Hindle, J. V., Jones, R. W., & Clare, L. (2019). The impact of co-morbidity on the quality of life of people with dementia: Findings from the IDEAL study. *Age and Ageing, 48*(3), 361–367.

O'Rourke, H. M., Duggleby, W., Fraser, K. D., & Jerke, L. (2015). Factors that affect quality of life from the perspective of people with dementia. *Ametasynthesis. Journal of the American Geriatrics Society, 63*(1), 24–38.

Palm, R., Trutschel, D., Sorg, C. G. G., Dichter, M. N., Haastert, B., & Holle, B. (2019). Quality of life in people with severe dementia and its association with the environment in nursing homes: An observational study. *Gerontologist, 59*(4), 665–674.

Phillips, K. (2016). Prescription writing; long term care; antipsychotic agents; Alzheimer's & dementia. *The Journal of the Alzheimer's Association, 12*(7), 263–264.

Schwarz, J., & Begley, S. (2003). *The mind & the brain.* Harper Collins.

Shamy, E. (1997). *More than body, brain and breath: A guide to spiritual care of people with Alzheimer's disease*. ColCom Press.

Szczepura, A., Wild, D., Khan, A. J., Owen, D. W., Palmer, T., Muhammad, T., Clark, M. D., & Bowman, C. (2016). Anti-psychotic prescribing in care homes before and after launch of a national dementia strategy: An observational study in English institutions over a four-year period. *British Medical Journal, Open*. Retrieved from https://bmjopen.bmj.com/

Wilkins, J. (2017). Dementia, decision making and quality of life. *American Medical Association Journal of Ethics*, *19*(7), 637–639.

Wilkinson, N., Srikumar, S., Shaw, K., & Orrell, M. (1998). Drama and movement therapy in dementia: A pilot study. *The Arts in Psychotherapy*, *2*(3), 195–201.

Chapter 5

Intelligence of feeling and dramatherapy

The qualitative research covered in the previous chapter has been useful in exploring some of the responses of individuals in the sessions recorded in the earlier Chapters 2 and 3, which show their willingness to share their life stage experiences in Chapter 2 and their fears about their diagnoses in Chapter 3. In the present chapter, my awareness of what I have called their "intelligence of feeling" (IoF) is defined and the case is made as to how this attribute of people with dementia can be heightened and identified in work using the arts, and dramatherapy in particular. When heart and mind are engaged (Verity & Lee, 2011) through the application of embodied movement (Jones, 2009), the experience makes a definitive difference. For example, in a vignette from Levy's work recorded by Jones, the dramatherapist reports that with her clients' work "embodying it allows her to get in touch with her emotions" (Jones, 2009, p. 100) as opposed to verbalising how she feels. Case examples of IoF recorded in dramatherapy sessions for my study are explored below, as well as a session where the IoF is observable in a reflection on objects provided. The EPR method (Jennings, 1999) is explained as a developmental intervention for all ages and reversed for the later life stages as Role, Projection and Embodiment (RPE). With the help of this method, the case is made for the promotion of feeling intelligence in people with dementia. EPR is also explained as a developmental intervention for all ages and reversed (RPE) for the late life stages.

Defining the intelligence of feeling

IoF is understood to be a sense of empathy towards the self and one's own feelings and memories, which can sometimes include others. It is distinguished here from emotion. Mulligan and Scherer (2012) reserve the term "emotion" for "short-lived affective episodes" (p. 347) and "feeling" as having an ability to communicate a subjective experience, thus possessing a governing function of the experience itself. Emotion revealed in psychotherapy often presents clients with a binary between effective and ineffective

DOI: 10.4324/9781003186328-5

emotions (David et al., 2004; Ellis, 1994). Insofar as we are aware, feelings have intelligence, and need to be taken seriously. Panhofer et al. suggest:

> that we are able to passively and actively experience within our relational world as wide and deep a set of feelings as both we and our relational world can bear. The relationship between feeling and emotion helps to clarify, with the former denoting individual subjective sensory and bodily experience and the latter implying the expression in the presence of others of the feeling.
>
> (2014, p. 117)

It is argued here though, that elders with dementia possess a more refined ability than usually recognised, which can transcend both the amalgamating and the binary antithesis of feeling (Jaaniste, 2013a). IoF (Jaaniste, 2013a) communicated by people with dementia includes memory and consciousness, in contrast to common deterioration in the frontal cortex of such people. Neuroscience informs us that the development of these elements in the unborn infant can inform us of problems taking place in later life (Gerhardt, 2015). Labar et al. (2000) report that the neural systems responsible for feeling–attention interactions are generated in the amygdala, deeper in the brain than the frontal cortex. This is an area which may have been passed over by researchers in the past because of an inappropriate emphasis on the higher cortex, thus neglecting cortex and subcortex.

Witkin (1974) believes that a sense of soul in the feeling life is "the inner act of reciprocation that lies at the heart of the creative movement" (p. 188). Sardello states that the feeling life is where the individuality is most present. "Feeling is that soul region where life first crosses over into experience" (2008, p. 55). When people with dementia are in a safe and contained group and feel valued and are allowed to express these feelings creatively, they show us who they really are (Jaaniste, 2013b).

IoF and memory

May et al. (2005) refer to research that suggests that in older age groups, there are only moderate age-related changes in the amygdala compared with other brain areas (Smith et al., 1999). They also find that although memory diminishes as people age, recall of "emotionally meaningful material" (May et al., 2005, p. 577) is relatively unimpaired. Sattler et al. (2007) found that in 20 subjects with Alzheimer's disease (AD) hearing a stimulating story with emotional content, there was more recall afterwards than in the control group of elders with no dementia. Thomaz et al. (2007) state that an increase in emotional motivation can be related to the concept of the IoF. Zeisel and Raia's (2000) awareness of a connection between the amygdala and AD was one of the first instances of this link.

The results of their investigation suggest that this area of the brain is one of the last to be affected by AD, remaining "readily accessible until very late in the disease" (Zeisel & Raia, 2000, p. 7).

Culturally, it seems likely that the IoF is stifled considerably if people are not met by "feeling language" (Kitwood, 1997, p. 79) or opportunities for "a multiplicity of feeling structures" (Harding & Pribram, 2002, p. 418). Dramatherapy, as a creative arts therapy, can be helpful in encouraging and allowing the expression of feeling. Rubin, in her foreword to Rappaport's focusing-oriented art text, mentions the "quiet inner listening … inviting the client to stop, listen, feel, look at and then express ideas, feelings and images from within" (Rapaport, 2009, p. 14). She considers dance-movement therapy as well as dramatherapy to be in this category. Such opportunities are presented in each of these modalities when reflection takes place after movement. An example of the quiet listening and feeling expression comes from a session which will be reported at the end of this chapter. After energetic warm-ups, Ben (73) was given a dirty crystalline rock to handle, which it was suggested he could transform from a symbol of fear into something more positive. He looked at it carefully and said: "once they're cleaned and all that, it's amazing. So there are things to look at, including your age". His use of metaphor is powerful – he is naming the fact that the fear needs "cleaning" or changing into a different feeling. He seems perhaps to be telling us that when we age, some things don't feel as scary anymore.

Dramatherapy and IoF

Like the other arts therapies, dramatherapy offers its art form using theatre and drama processes for the purpose of healing. Approaches such as roleplay, improvisation, embodiment and voice work, puppetry and mask making are available for clients to express themselves. Interventions are offered aiming for client expression of inner challenges as well as celebratory emotions to enable participants to face significant issues in their daily lives (Jaaniste, 2013a; 2013b).

The dramatherapy space can be thought of as a safe playing space for the entire range of human feelings for people with dementia. For many of them, there are opportunities to share challenging responses to visits from family members, which may be rare opportunities or may not occur at all. They may wish to save their families anxiety, or if they are in a care home, understaffing may affect quality time spent with carers. In her heuristic exploration of her own experience of working with a group of older adults with dementia, dramatherapist Morris (2011) finds words for the joy she and her clients experience in the dramatherapy group, where they may also express the fear and anxiety associated with the disease and its diagnosis. This is a necessity not only for clients but for herself as a therapist: "Dementia gradually takes hold of people, suffocating their abilities, personality and memories. This is a terrifying concept and fear itself has become an essential component of my research" (2011, p. 148).

Then, a personal note from her research log:

> I am now in touch with the fear attached to the diagnosis of dementia. It seems to exist on a cultural and personal level … stirred even by close friends and family. Dramatherapy can perhaps work with this often unconscious fear, by offering unconditional positive regard, respect, acceptance and encouragement.
>
> (Log, August 2010) (Morris, 2011, pp. 148–149)

Qualified dramatherapists are trained to undertake the essential role described by Morris, providing a safe space for the participants, witnessing a broad range of feelings. Various interventions can be chosen to facilitate this process in different ways. Sue Jennings' EPR method (Jennings, 1999) is a safe way to allow the clients to express themselves. In this method, activities of embodying a feeling, projecting onto an object or taking on a role synchronise with the early developmental process of the human being. Awareness of the sequencing of interventions in this process is an essential ingredient for therapists to enable the engagement of clients gradually and naturally into a trustful group experience. The explanation below of the developmental aspects of the method includes information on how it can be reversed and used to advantage with people with dementia.

Embodiment, Projection and Role

EPR techniques are useful for the dramatherapist in choosing the means to assist diverse populations to fulfil their goals in the dramatherapy space. These three different kinds of interventions can be used for assessment purposes, linking with the milestones in early development. They can be even more powerful if the history of the client is shared or known from an early age. It is possible to engage clients by using these techniques in either individual or group dramatherapy. It became clear to me once I began to work with elderly people and especially those with dementia that Jennings' (1999, pp. 51–53) order could be reversed, as mentioned above. This reversal offers the opportunity to find ways to use the method with older people so that it fulfils the needs of their life stage (Jaaniste, 2016; Jennings, 1999). In 2016, Sue Jennings spoke to me in an interview about the EPR method: "It shows the power of drama to enable hypothesis and discovery" (Jaaniste, 2016, pp. 89–90). She went on to say that additional practice and observance of the method, together with advances in neuroscience, helped her to develop her work in Neuro-Dramatic Play, which concentrates on the earliest stage of EPR. In contrast, my reversal of the paradigm engages with the other end of the life cycle (Jaaniste, 2016).

Embodiment: These interventions for embodiment issues involve engaging the client somatically. This involves gradual facial expression, bodily gesture and paced limb movement as long as the client can achieve this without pain or discomfort. These non-cognitive exercises can assist clients by degrees where there may have been disturbing past bodily experiences, to permit touch and gain somatic self-awareness. These interventions are not among those used initially with a client, but are introduced gradually over time, as safety and trust-building are paramount for the strengthening of client confidence in their own embodied identity as individuals (Jaaniste, 2018).

When we observe a very young baby's movements, we see fingers curling, feet waving and facial expressions changing from moment to moment. Infants move and play along with their environment physically, in order to experience it. This flailing and rippling, and later rolling and twisting, helps them to connect with their surroundings and develop identity later on. For the older adults in my research, there is the opportunity to warm-up, as described in Chapter 3, and to revisit early memories – the first ones laid down and the last to be forgotten. They often need assistance to participate through the demonstration of the dramatherapist and support workers, as well as from video.

Projection: Projective interventions increase the development of the client's imagination, providing symbolic objects which can become metaphors for exploring lived experience so far and hopes for change. By exploring concrete objects and toys, or making art to provide a client's own images, relationships to others and to his own story can be established.

Here the child relates more to the outer world, beyond his body. There is a focus on the objects and toys belonging to his environment. During this stage, children explore the world through their own relationships to objects, and stories can be dramatised through toys, dolls or other objects. It is often easier for them to speak of their own needs through those of their teddy bear or favourite doll, for example: "Teddy wants a blanket".

Role: Role-play as an intervention is a means of assisting the client to find unexpected connections with the self and others. Taking on a role, no matter how different that role is from the client's perceived everyday self, can bring important realisations about the nature of the self, the over-used role she plays in life or a new aspect of a role she would like to add to her collection. For example, a high-status role may bring the realisation there is more need for authority in her voice or bearing.

The toddler changes at about three years old when the child identifies herself as "I". Dramatic play becomes a new way of being, and she starts to distinguish between everyday and dramatic reality as she plays familiar and unfamiliar roles. Role-modelling coming from parents and caregivers is played out. The child borrows the caregiver's clothes and "en-roles".

Role, Projection and Embodiment

The sequence of this paradigm has been reversed by the author for elders because, especially for people with dementia, taking on a role is easier for those whose dementia is at a mild level, as at this stage, they know the difference between "me" and "not me". Projection works best for people in a moderate state of dementia, as their thinking is more concrete at this stage, and embodiment is successful when the person has a severe diagnosis of the disease, since body language can take over when words fail them. Embodiment can be mirrored by the group in games, demonstrated as mentioned above, or connected with a theme. If the theme is The Weather, for example, as in Session 1, they are asked to move as though blown about by the wind or swimming in the surf. The use of the method in this way has nothing to do with infantilisation. Infantilisation is a destructive treatment of older people, quoted by Kitwood as a "malignant social psychology" (1997, p. 45). An awareness of social psychology with integrity is essential when connecting with people who may have one or more experiences such as intense anxiety, feelings of abandonment, betrayal, confusion or boredom, sometimes caused by well-intended but uninformed family or carers (Kitwood, 1997, p. 79).

Feeling and emotion

Behaviourist traditions, which have regarded acting, thinking and feeling as "behaviours" based on reaction rather than reflection or any warmth of sensibility (Baum, 2005), have influenced binary thinking. This type of thinking privileges cognition over perceptive and thoughtful command of emotional reaction. IoF, on the other hand, is a subtle and filtered ability which involves memory and consciousness (Gerhardt, 2015) and can emanate from people with dementia. IoF is connected to the heart and soul, as de St. Exupéry points out: "It is only with the heart that one can see rightly; what is essential is invisible to the eye" (1995, p. 82).

When we look for the "intelligence of feeling" we are asking questions regarding emotional regulation rather than reactive responses to difficult situations. We are also not subscribing to the thesis that thinking and the self are completely bound together (Kontos, 2012; Kontos & Martin, 2013). Some research indicates that if a parent shows empathy when children become emotional, the children become more flexible within circumstances that have caused this state, and are more likely to display reflective skills once they become adults (Denham, 1998; Lievegoed, 1997). The heart centre opens to a feeling sense. Neurocardiologists investigating the relationship between brain and heart throw light on this connection. Direct and indirect association between brain and heart have been found to be present by Thayer and Lane (2009) through neuroimaging procedures. These neurophysiologists inform us that to approach feeling intelligence, observation is not enough and heart feeling needs to be taken into account, as well as cognitive abilities (Jaaniste, 2013b).

Neil – Case study

Neil, at 62 with early onset dementia, was the youngest of the group of participants in the fieldwork. He was somewhat non-committal about joining the programme from the first invitation to participate in the dramatherapy group. His partner was able to consider Neil's independence of thought, and because of her respect for his agency, he was not being pressured to join (Jaaniste, 2013a).

Overall, reluctant or not, Neil could not help himself from taking initiative and modelling highly socialised behaviour. He was very encouraging to others and open about his feelings throughout the 16 sessions, and this honest approach paid dividends for him as others strove to connect with him. A group often needs such a "communicator" in the dynamic, and once Neil had started to feel comfortable in the group after a few sessions, he appeared to want to maximise others' performance in the group and not just his own.

In the very first session of the program, it is important to find the right stimulus. A large number of black and white photographs were offered to the clients so that they could choose one which attracted their attention. Connecting with and reflecting on an image in a therapeutic context can promote the development of "epistemic trust" within the therapeutic relationship (Buck & Havsteen-Franklin, 2013). In this instance, it assisted in warming up the clients. Neil chose a hang-gliding picture. I asked him if he had done any hang-gliding. He replied in the negative, and then informed us that he was "a heavy sort of person, not as in weight but as in …" and was unable to finish this sentence. I wondered if he meant that he saw himself as prone to heavy moods, and he thought the suggestion came close to the sense he wanted to impart. He had chosen the picture because hang-gliding was an activity that lifted one's mood, with the understanding that it was a polar opposite to his own sense of self. Already he was presenting with a feeling sense of wanting to engage with the image, despite his initial reluctance to join.

Nevertheless, the heaviness was present for at least the first four sessions. It was easy to understand why. As he was the person with dementia in its mildest form, the people around him seemed weird and he said so. Yet he had a feeling of intelligence connected with a lively imagination. In Session 3 – Finding Treasure – he picked out a candle with an angelic message from the object bag. C. G. Jung's (1951) understanding of symbol used by his clients was deeply entwined with a here-and-now attention to his patient's symbols "and to areas of collapsed imagination, opening the image by listening to it differently", as pointed out by Butler (2016, p. 52). Butler goes on to say that in understanding the psyche as image, Jung came up with a therapeutic method which prioritises the relationship to images in their familiar environment: the imagination (Butler, 2016). When questioned about the object, Neil reported "a sense of being ... I have been blessed". When asked what he believed about its reference to angels, he said: "Not the floaty ones ... but um spirits, who um, sort of go with you".

Neil had a strong sense of social justice and displayed feeling intelligence in Session 4 when the group made art works as warm-ups to improvisation. Neil was silent while painting, finally showing us a new national flag he had designed, completed with dot-painting in blue and white (see Figure 5.1). The dot points were made as a reference to our Indigenous people, in recognition that they are not represented on the Australian National flag. Paul, who had a strong sense of justice also, asked, "What about the First People?" I asked Neil if he would like to use the flag as a starting point for a group performance, and he agreed to do so. I had already promised Tanya, early in the session, that we would find a time for her to stamp her feet. (She felt like doing so, as she was frustrated that she could not remember who had brought her to the session that morning.) He continued to encourage the group to be strong (a favourite adjective) and there was a consensus that they should make a performance about marching in protest about the lack of authenticity

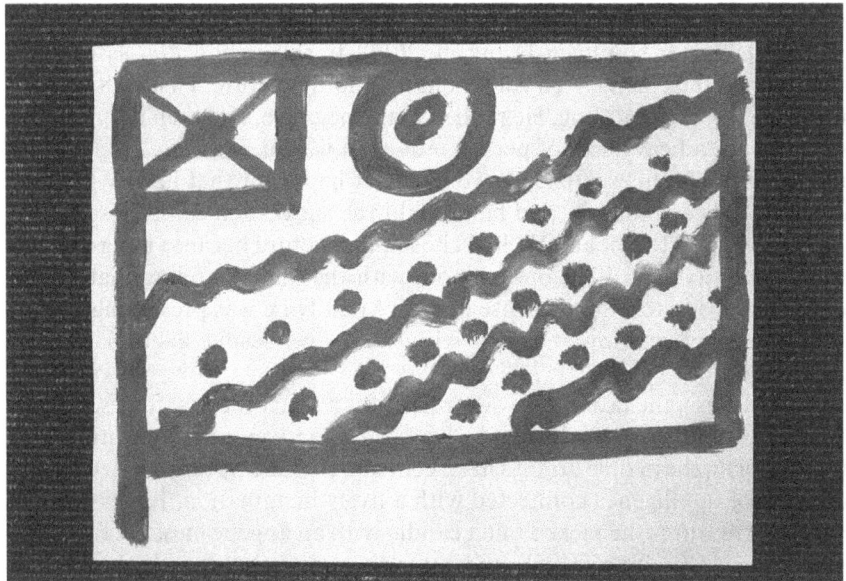

Figure 5.1 Neil's Australian flag

of our present flag. Soon they had chosen a staff member to be prime minister, and I asked them to choose names for themselves so that they could de-role from their protesting selves later.[1] In no time, they were "in Canberra" with Neil leading the line of protesters to Parliament House, encouraging participants to wave imaginary flags and shouting: "We want to change the flag" (Jaaniste, 2013a).

On arrival at "Parliament House", the Prime Minister (Tony Abbott at the time) asked Neil, as spokesperson, why they wanted to change the flag. This was his reply:

> A lot of, a lot of Australians think that they need to change the flag ... there needs to be a consensus. And politicians don't believe in – well often don't believe in, ah, consensus. Thank you. Thank you very much. Politicians don't often believe in consensus so this is, this is part of the process. It's not the end of things. It's just part of the process.

Neil had showed strong IoF for his fellow Australians and their exclusion from the democratic process by cheering them on and displaying empathy. He had tried to get Paul to be the PM, saying he would be "a good man for the job", but Paul was not willing. Then he had said to the staff member: "Well I'll get my friend over here. She's a solid citizen". Then to David: "Do you want to stand up and march with me? Ok? So we're going up to the Parliament House. You've got to join in now".

It was also interesting that there was a metaphor here of protesting and fighting for the national flag to include others, at exactly the same time as Alzheimer's Australia was using the slogan "Fight Dementia" and conducting protest walks with carers and others to raise awareness of the disease and the effect it had on elderly Australians. The idea of protesting also came into the session which I identified as the "storming" phase of the group, in Tuckman's (1965) and Yalom's (1995) terms. The resistance that typically happens in this phase was able to be incorporated into the intervention.

In Session 6, when the group was involved in Developmental Transformations (DvT), and the Magic Box stage of the intervention became an Emotional Soup where participants could improvise throwing in any unwanted issues, Neil threw in the anger of men who did not have access to their children. On the way to the session that day his carer had driven him across the Sydney Harbour Bridge where a man was demonstrating from a precarious height on behalf of separated or divorced fathers who had no custody of their children. I wondered if this was about the children in his life (his nieces and nephews) who he said did not visit him. Neil did not have children of his own; he had plenty of empathy though for fathers and this showed itself in his facial expression and tone of voice. He said later in session that he and his wife, who had both married late in life, made a decision not to have children. There were perhaps anxieties within Neil about the future – would nieces and nephews visit if and when dementia debilitated him further?

In Session 8, when the participants were celebrating themselves just before the break of a fortnight, Neil told Leanne what he thought about her artistic talents, and Katsuko, one of the art therapy students, told him about his frankness and honesty and then she admitted to sometimes feeling afraid. This prompted a disclosure from Neil that was touching and showed feeling intelligence. He very shyly reported as follows: "I get embarrassed, because I think other people know more, or have got more, or whatever, but I don't; but, here, it's like, a very easy place to be. You can be as silly as you like". When he added the following, he used a stronger tone: "It's important for me to remember what I can do rather than what I can't do now. You know, I can't do a lot of things now, and I need to remind myself that once I was able to" (Jaaniste, 2013b). Katsuko said that Neil had been brave enough to say what many of us feel at times in our lives and he didn't treat the tribute with denial as others are prone to do. His dialogue here can also be seen as a reference to the fact that the elderly often need to be reminded of who they once were, together with talents and abilities they may no longer have. He also used "I" to describe his abilities, whereas most people are not good at this. His background as a counsellor may have assisted him with the language of "I" rather than "you".

In Session 9, we played a game of Statues where participants walked around the room and took on a frozen statuesque position when I clapped twice. Neil shared in the reflection at the end of the session that when he was moving around, apparently aimlessly, there was a memory which returned to him from when he was in Year 10 at school. He was caned by a teacher for transferring basketballs from a storeroom to the outdoor courts for the benefit of some more junior students at the lunch break. "It would have been different if I had been jumping in and out of windows", he said. His was an example of the memories of unfairness that can come with dementia, like Leanne's which was mentioned in Chapter 2.

When I asked Neil if this memory gave him the chance to experience an empathic response to Leanne's story, he explained that the two situations were different; he said this was a remembrance of one occasion only, whereas Leanne's was "constant torture". Neil said the memory had come up for a reason – "something that was dead and buried – 45 years or something". I had provided them with hats to wear if they chose, to facilitate past memories, and he told us his hat was the trigger – a baseball cap worn back to front. It encouraged him to "kick the paintwork, to stomp around a bit and be a bit stroppy". Apparently, the cap was the kind of hat he would have worn to school.

Tian Dayton comments on qualities of psychodrama which assist a gradual movement from activity to resolution, which could equally be seen as a description of movement accompanied by simple dressups in drama-therapy. The activity had enabled a clear distinction between Neil's feeling and Leanne's, while at the same time acknowledging the complexity of her trauma as differing from his own experience:

> The beauty of exploring the emotion through action is that the emotion can surface as originally felt, and can be explored from that perspective first – before it is edited or reflected upon in any way. This is a process of joining and moving into a person's inner reality, of validating it as it exists within that person, with no attempt to manipulate it to conform to other people's perceptions.
>
> (Dayton, 1994, p. 2)

There are features of Session 7 on grief and loss and of Session 14, entitled Past, present and future, when Neil showed examples of feeling intelligence. These descriptions, however, are to be found in Chapters 7, 8 and 9, which deal with grief in old age, trauma and intersubjectivity, and the mystery of death. For the purposes of this case study, however, Neil's feeling intelligence came to the fore in these three areas, and especially in his support of Leanne's work on her very deep-seated recognition of complex trauma from her childhood. In Session 12, he was able to say he felt "at home" finally in the group. This greater confidence in his participation came to the fore in Session 13 when he told of a childhood memory of floating in the river on the inner tube of an old tyre. It was the first time he had ever floated, and he remarked: "It was just an amazing moment and it was scary but I loved it". He stood and watched as other members of the group improvised this experience for him, and said, "Don't drown". This appeared to be a metaphor for "hang in there, as I have done. You may end up by free-floating".

In the program's last session, Neil was more silent than usual. When it came to talking about the session being the last, he reported feeling a hollowness, that it would take some time for him to connect with people again. He did acknowledge the relationships he had established, particularly through the group singing at the end of each session – "I love that we threw the ball to one another and voiced the qualities we would miss about the program". He chose, "play", "company", "a mixture of joy and sadness" and "laughter".

A dramatherapy session honouring the IoF

This was Session 12 in the series and it was the meeting where unexpected IoF was the most observable, heightened by the poetic nature of metaphor. The title of the session is The land of forgetfulness, so it is ironic that so much of this ability was displayed in a meeting about memory loss.

During our opening chat, when I was introducing them to the idea of memory and its loss, the following conversation took place:

PAUL: Yes, I discovered a lot of things about memory, or lack of memory.
JOANNA: Yes? What have you discovered?
PAUL: Well I forget things left, right, and centre. Forgotten.
LYNNE: Gone, gone, gone, gone, gone.
NOEL: Very good. Ah, good one.
PAUL (85, with Parkinsonism and moderate dementia) rubbed his head: I used to have a lot of hair here … and then it became smooth and then it became all spotty.

Our first warm-up in the session was Fruit Bowl (Farmer, 2007, p. 3) and the second was Adam and Eve (Scher & Verrall, 1975, p. 24). The first was chosen for the hilarity caused by participants mis-remembering if they had been named an apple, an orange or a banana. The second was chosen because it involved a blindfolded "Adam", so that the participant playing him needed to follow the voice of "Eve" and remember where they had heard it last in an attempt to tag the voice of participant playing Eve. A similar scenario was played out with Eve looking for Adam. During the game, Paul suddenly announced that he had a story to tell us, as follows:

> Well, my daughter wrote a book and her book was about architecture and children, because children can get into a state where they fall in a building because they don't know it's there or because it's badly placed, or something like that, and so they do that and I have said to my daughter she should not have done that for children. You should have done that with grandparents. Grandparents would be saved the troubles. That's the story.

Paul's story seems important here, firstly because Paul had been an architect himself and his story links him professionally with his daughter, and secondly because it is a touching reminder of his Parkinsonism with its accompanying unsteadiness. The additional blindfolding brought an element of the uncomfortable reality of his physical disability, otherwise unmentioned by him, into the room. It also brings in the awareness of his life stage as a grandparent and highlights his constructive and regenerative concerns.

Since the game had proved useful to the clients, I took a further risk and asked everyone to get down on the floor and increase physical closeness even further. Everyone linked arms and placed their hands palms down, so that no pair of hands were next to each other but instead alternated with those of the participants on either side of them. Then I patted the floor to demonstrate and each hand needed to pat it in turn, taking account of the fact that each person had another's hand between their own pair. It was a hilarious game as people made mistakes at first and finally found a rhythm. They had built up a trust over time and this had assisted them to tolerate mistakes. The humour served as an entrée to "magical space".

The next intervention was to build the DvT space that we made in Session 6, The joys and woes of memory, which is described in Chapter 2. (Please refer to Chapter 3, pp. 34–35 for the description of the Magic Box, one of the techniques within this method [Johnson, 1986; Sandel & Johnson, 1987]). I initiated this again as it had worked well a few weeks previously, and also because I wanted to make the main activity of the day seem special. The whole intervention used some of the ideas put forward by Macy and Brown (1998) and is called The Truth Mandala.

These two authors explain how this ritual exercise offers an uncomplicated group structure in order to give respect to our suffering for the world. The intervention was born in 1992 in a vast gathering that was filled with tension in Frankfurt on Reunification Day between West and East Germany, and it has since spread to many other countries throughout the world (Macy & Brown, 1998). My clinical supervisor suggested it as a means to help transform individual losses from the past such as failing memory abilities, which were being revealed by participants.

Once we had walked around the room and limbered up in our bodies, we climbed into the imaginary play space, then sat in a circle, close together, forming a container for the transformative experiences that were hopefully coming towards us. In each quadrant of the circle, there were placed symbolic objects: stones, dead leaves and petals, sticks and bowls. I explained to the participants that each group of objects had a certain meaning. I paraphrased the words the authors used to describe their symbolism:

> The stone is for fear. It is how our heart feels when we're afraid: tight, contracted, hard.
> These dry leaves represent our sorrow, our grief. There is great sadness within us from what we see happening in our world, our lives, and for what is passing from us.
> The stick is for our anger. For there is anger and outrage in us that needs to be spoken for clarity of mind and purpose. This stick is not for hitting with or waving around, but for grasping hard with our hands – it's strong enough for that.
> And in this fourth quadrant, the empty bowl stands for our sense of deprivation and need, our hunger for what's missing, our emptiness.
> (Macy & Brown, 1998, pp. 101–102)

These objects were presented to the participants as an opportunity to transform some of the feelings that are linked with unwanted forgetfulness, and it was made clear to them that they could take items from each quadrant of the circle with their suggested meanings (Jaaniste, 2013a). They worked in dyads once they had chosen, exchanging views on what the objects meant to them, finally joining the group and reflecting on the objects together.

In DvT, there are generally no concrete objects available within the space of the Magic Box, nor verbal reflection after the drama. In a personal communication with David Johnson, however, he told me that he occasionally uses objects there to stimulate the imaginations of participants. We were both aware that projection was particularly important to these people, as most had moderate dementia which coincides with the importance of projection in RPE. Group reflection time was outside the playspace, and Johnson is fine with this method, despite its variation from the usual stages of his DvT intervention (Johnson, personal communication, March 17, 2012).

Once we had formed the circle, pulled down the curtain and stepped through it, we sat down next to one another and I gave the following instructions:

> So come back into a circle – a little bit bigger. And now we're going to have to shut our eyes whilst something else happens. So turning around – so if you can turn around – so that we back onto the circle and shut your eyes. It's going to take a little while for this to be organised. So if you can just stay there with your eyes shut for a few minutes please. Something's going to happen in the circle. You might be thinking about some time in your life when you had to shut your eyes and some surprise was happening. Thank you all for being so patient. Now you can turn slowly around and in our magic circle there are some special things today, but we've first of all we've got to make this place very safe so we all put our hands up and pull down the curtain. Pull it right down to the floor. Then part – when you get up, part the curtain. So there'll be a split in the curtain right in front of you. So part the curtain and step into the play space and pull the curtain behind you. Now we're in the circle – pull the curtain behind you.
>
> Open your eyes ... Now we're in a safe play space and here in our play space there are some symbols. So what do you make of them? There's some anger, some fear, some tears, and some emptiness. Maybe this is all to do with the land of forgetfulness. What do people make of all that? Maybe just set this out a little differently so it's not such a chunk.

Once people opened their eyes, Ben immediately said, "There seems to be more to play with. I've got four kids and ... these are made from that place and if you don't get that sort of material up there then they're not – they're not happy". It seemed to me that Ben's inner child was ready to work with the surprise, and later on, he mentioned Christmas.

Participants worked in pairs, and staff members and trainee art therapists helped people to understand the instructions. When everyone was still working in their dyads within the play space, Neil said it was nice to talk to someone. Paul was interested to compare two objects, the stick (he had a Japanese chopstick) and a stone. Leanne joined into the comparison, and found that her stone was heavy and her leaves and petals were light. Ben told us the tears were definitely not his, but he started to talk about someone who was crying. Paul, Neil and Ben had a conversation between the three of them – most unusually, as in our sessions, people normally spoke either one to one or to the whole group in general.

PAUL: Those two are close to
NEIL: A gentle place.
BEN: It is. That's indeed a fact.
PAUL: Interesting and close to each other.
JOANNA: Close to each other.
PAUL: As a pair.
JOANNA: As a pair.
PAUL: Mm.

There seemed to be a metaphorical recognition among these people that they were drawing closer to each other, in the light of the very human qualities and values we were discussing.

We moved out of the play space at this stage, taking the chosen objects with us. I shared what the objects meant to me in their transformed state. Ben shared that his stone looked like a stalactite: "There's very blue stalactites like that not so long ago. On the floor, that is. That happens when you get around. That sort of thing. Eyes prickly – sort of space". It seemed that the idea of crying might be affecting him after all. He continued: "once they're cleaned and all that, it's amazing ... So there are things to look at, including your age". It seemed as though Ben, whose moderate dementia was becoming severe, might be telling us something about clearing a space for looking at old age.

In the playspace, Leanne had said her stone was heavy; however, once outside in the group circle, she told us that her stone of fear had another quality, as she showed us "that magnificent chunk of splendour".

LEANNE: It's beautiful, it's endurable ... It's intriguing, because it's got a brown stripe around it, and when you come to the top, it's beautifully sparkled all over. So there's something hidden somewhere.
PAUL: The sparkles wouldn't be there if it wasn't for that *(indicating the dull brown foundation of the rock)*.

This seemed to be a wise, quasi-Jungian point about finding gold in the shadow (Johnson, 1991). Then Leanne continued in aesthetic mode that could well be noted by the architects and designers of retirement villages (Jaaniste, 2013a):

LEANNE: *(dreamily)* It's beautiful ... we need to see beauty, because if we don't see it, something dies in us ... you've got to search for the good stuff, and it's always a joy to see it ... incredible, isn't it, it grows from that stuff *(pointing to the brown stripe)* to that stuff *(pointing out the sparkling amethyst crystal)*.

Neil showed us his collection of petals, and then spoke to us:

NEIL: *(filled with feeling)* I was seeing beauty in the flowers, and I was thinking, 'Oh, that's nice', and then all of a sudden I just felt tears and then we started talking about ...
JOANNA: What were the tears about?
NEIL: Oh, the sadness of family issues, death of parents, mm ...

Ben showed everyone a stone he had chosen, and used what appeared to be a metaphor for this wearying dis-ease and requiring assistance with his dementia:

BEN: I can't give it any more, other than someone who can clean the thing up again and give it some shine.

Paul had picked up a chopstick as mentioned earlier, and this recalled for him, rather than anger, the Japanese cultural significance for his family, while at the same time almost certainly acknowledging art therapy student Katsuko:

PAUL: One of my sons married a Japanese girl, and she brought new thinking, forms of thinking, and so did the fathers and uncles and so forth ... the Japanese connections have been very strong, and very, very much appreciated by me *(broad smile)*.

There was conversation about experiencing fear when growing up, yet not engendering it in one's own children by one staff member, and seeing a mother lose her memory through dementia by another. Paul spoke of "a sort of feeling of humanity and the possible worth of humanity and the possible continuation of humanity" and Ben of "certain touches and tastes of the music", even though we had not yet ended with a song, which we always did. Neil shared, "I think I feel at home here ... which means that I wasn't before". It really seemed as though the transformation of the sticks, stones, petals and bowls had brought value to the participants.

Poignantly, I had selected a piece of petrified wood from among the stones of fear: a fear of losing my own memory as my mother had for some years before she died. My fear had been transformed though by the privilege of working with these participants, sharing their aesthetic sense of wonder – their sense of loss too – but strong gratitude for what remained with them.

This session gave me the strongest sense of the participants' IoF. It would not, I believe, have been possible to work with a transformational ritual of such a high order if the interpersonal trust in the group had not been as strong. Because of this generous spirit and feeling sense shared in the group, it was possible to introduce the ritual at this stage. Sajnani (2012) calls this "feeling sense" when associated with improvisation, and I identify it as connected with IoF. She believes:

> Improvisation promotes aesthetic intelligence by heightening one's attention to one's senses, to others and to when 'it' is 'working'. George Steiner has commented that we do not have a word yet for this 'ordered enlistment of intuition' (1989: 12). Indeed, improvisation involves the development of sophisticated skills *and* an intuitive responsiveness to the unexpected.
>
> (Sajnani, 2012, p. 83)

It is evident that participants need to be approached on their own levels, however sophisticated the concepts used in our sessions. It is also essential to have an awareness of metaphor and the potential meaning behind their words, in order to engage participants' consciousness. A consideration of their IoF needs to be present, and the soul life of the people with dementia needs to be considered in all the arts therapies. As Sardello points out:

> the phenomena of soul life are available to consciousness and can be described ... it becomes necessary to be able to speak from within what one is observing; that is to say, the observer is inevitably an aspect of what one observes when working from a soul perspective.
>
> (2008, pp. 7–8)

The next chapter will consider technology and artificial intelligence (AI) and the role they are beginning to play in the care of older people. The discussion of their relevance in bringing dramatherapy to elders and people with dementia is one that needs to consider the ethical implications of working with telehealth and incorporating technological interventions into the arts therapy space.

Note

1 De-roling "has a function to assist the player to leave the role and return to their normal reality" (Jones 2007, p. 216). The dramatherapist usually encourages an en-roled participant to shake their body thoroughly, de-identifying themselves from the character they have played, and stating their own name.

References

Baum, W. (2005). *Understanding behaviourism* (2nd ed.). Blackwell.

Buck, E. T., & Havsteen-Franklin, D. (2013). Connecting with the image: How psychotherapy can help to re-establish a sense of epistemic trust. *Art Therapy Online, 4*(1), 1.

Butler, J. (2016). Gnawing at the roots: Towards a transpersonal poetics of guilt and death. *International Journal of Transpersonal Studies, 35*(2), 50–60.

David, D., Montgomery, G. H., Macavei, B., & Bovbjerg, D. H. (2004). An empirical investigation of Albert Ellis' binary model of distress. *Journal of Clinical Psychology, 61*(4), 499–516.

Dayton, T. (1994). *The drama within: Psychodrama and experiential therapy*. Health Communications, Inc.

Denham, S. (1998). *Emotional development in young children*. Guilford Press.

de Saint-Exupéry, A. (1995). *The little prince*. Wordsworth Editions.

Ellis, A. (1994). *Reason and emotion in psychotherapy: Comprehensive method of treating human disturbances* (Rev. ed.). Citadel Press.

Farmer, D. (2007). *101 drama games and activities*. Lulu Press.

Gerhardt, S. (2015). *Why love matters* (2nd ed.). Routledge.

Harding, J., & Pribram, E. D. (2002). The power of feeling: Locating emotions in culture. *European Journal of Cultural Studies, 5*(4), 407–426.

Jaaniste, J. (2013a). The intelligence of feeling and dramatherapy with people with dementia. In S. Petruzzella, M. Ross, & S. Scoble (Eds.), *Arts therapies and the intelligence of feeling* (pp. 117–130). University of Plymouth Press.

Jaaniste, E. J. (2013b). *Pulled through a hedge backwards: Improving the quality of life of people with dementia through dramatherapy* [Unpublished PhD Thesis]. University of Western Sydney.

Jaaniste, J. (2016). Interview with Sue Jennings. *Australian & New Zealand Journal of Arts Therapy, 11*(1), 87–93.

Jaaniste, J. (2018). Quality of life improvement through dramatherapy for people with dementia: A developmental approach. *Australian & New Zealand Journal of Arts Therapy, 13*(1 & 2), 77–82.

Jennings, S. (1999). *Introduction to developmental playtherapy*. Jessica Kingsley Publishers.

Johnson, D. (1986). The developmental method in dramatherapy: Group treatment with the elderly. *The Arts in Psychotherapy, 13*, 17–33.

Johnson, D. (1991). The theory and technique of transformations in drama therapy. *The Arts in Psychotherapy, 18*(4), 285–300.

Jones, P. (2007). *Drama as therapy: Theory, practice and research* (2nd ed.). Routledge.

Jones, P. (2009). Therapists' understandings of embodiment in dramatherapy: Findings from a research approach using vignettes and a MSN messenger research conversations. *Body Movement and Dance in Psychotherapy, 4*(2), 95–106.

Jung, C. G. (1951). In H. Read, M. Fordham, G. Adler, & W. McGuire (Eds.), *The collected works of C. G. Jung: Aion* (R. F. C. Hull, Trans., Vol. ii). Princeton University Press.

Kitwood, T. (1997). *Dementia reconsidered*. Open University Press.

Kontos, P. (2012). Rethinking sociability in long-term care: An embodied dimension of selfhood. *Dementia, 11*(3), 329–346.

Kontos, P., & Martin, W. (2013). Embodiment and dementia: Exploring critical narratives of selfhood, surveillance, and dementia care. *Dementia*, *12*(3), 288–302.

Labar, K. S., Mesulem, M., Gitelman, D. R., & Weintraub, S. (2000). Emotional curiosity: Modulation of visuospatial attention by arousal is preserved in aging and early stage Alzheimer's disease. *Neuropsychologia*, *38*, 1734–1740.

Lievegoed, B. (1997). *Phases: The spiritual rhythms in adult life*. Sophia Books.

Macy, J., & Brown, Y. (1998). *Coming back to life: Practices to reconnect our lives, our world*. New Society Publishers.

May, C., Rahhal, T., Berry, M., & Leighton, E. (2005). Aging, source memory and emotion. *Psychology and Aging*, *20*(4), 571–578.

Morris, N. (2011). Unspoken depths: Dramatherapy and dementia. *Dramatherapy*, *33*(3), 144–157.

Mulligan, K., & Scherer, K. R. (2012). Toward a working definition of emotion. *Emotion Review*, *4*(4), 457.

Panhofer, H., Garcia, M. E., & Zelaskowski, P. (2014). The challenge of working with the embodied mind in the context of a university-based dance-movement therapy program. *The Arts in Psychotherapy*, *41*, 115–119.

Rapaport, L. (2009). *Focusing-oriented art therapy: Accessing the body's wisdom and creative intelligence*. Jessica Kingsley.

Sajnani, N. (2012). Improvisation and art-based research. *Journal of Applied Arts and Health*, *3*(1), 79–86.

Sandel, S., & Johnson, D. (1987). *Waiting at the gate: Creativity & hope in the nursing home*. The Haworth Press.

Sardello, R. (2008). *Love and the soul*. Goldenstone Press.

Sattler, C., Garrido, L. M., Sarmiento, E. P., Leme, S., Conde, C., & Tomaz, C. (2007). Emotional arousal enhances declarative memory in patients with Alzheimer's disease. *Acta Neurologica*, *116*(6), 355–360.

Scher, A., & Verrall, C. (1975). *100+ ideas for drama*. Heinemann.

Smith, C. D., Malcein, M., Meurer, M., Schmitt, F. A., Markesberry, W. R., & Pettigrew, L. C. (1999). MRI temporal lobe volume measures and neuropsychologic function in Alzheimer's disease. *Journal of Neuroimaging*, *9*, 2–9.

Thayer, J., & Lane, R. (2009). Claude Bernard and the heart–brain connection: Further elaboration of a model of neurovisceral integration. *Neuroscience and Biobehavioural Reviews*, *33*, 81–88.

Thomaz, C. E., Duran, F. L., Busatto, G. F., Gillies, D. F., & Rueckert, D. (2007). Multivariate statistical differences of MRI samples of the human brain. *Journal of Mathematical Imaging and Vision*, *29*, 95–106.

Tuckman, B. W. (1965). Developmental sequence in small groups. *Psychological Bulletin*, *63*(5), 384–399.

Verity, J., & Lee, H. (2011). Reigniting the human spirit. In H. Lee, & T. Adams (Eds.), *Creative approaches in dementia care* (pp. 16–31). Palgrave MacMillan.

Witkin, R. (1974). *The intelligence of feeling*. Heinemann.

Yalom, I. D. (1995). *The theory and practice of group psychotherapy*. Basic Books.

Zeisel, J., & Raia, P. (2000). Non-pharmacological treatment for Alzheimer's disease: A mind-brain approach. *American Journal of Alzheimer's Disease and Other Dementias*, *15*(6), 331–340.

Chapter 6

The ethical debate about technology and artificial intelligence

In the previous chapter, people with dementia were found to be endowed with a special kind of intelligence of feeling which compensates to some extent for their difficulties in the cognitive realm. This unique sensitivity to the human condition, often expressed via metaphor, is closely associated with a sense of community and the possibility of energetic response and physical touch. There are so many ways in which the dramatherapist can inspire elders, individually or in groups, to take creative risks and express themselves in movement or through sound using approaches that are usually applied face to face. Some of these are increasingly being delivered through artificial intelligence (AI). Some possibilities in this area are very recent, and there are several questions for their use for people with dementia. There are many opportunities to use technology as well – especially video and sound systems which we are more familiar with. These will be explored in this chapter, along with the ethics of using AI when working with elderly people with dementia with creative arts therapies.

AI and robots in aged care

Robots have been replacing people since the 1960s and because of this, McGinn and his colleagues in Dublin have explored the proliferation of AI in the aged care sector (McGinn, 2017). The authors expect that robots will be taking on some of the routine tasks of looking after the elderly, including those with dementia. They hope this will leave human carers free to focus on the more personal parts of the job.

Certainly, McGinn's robots can remind the client to take medication, regulate room temperatures and deal with certain obstacles that could result in falls. They can also organise a Skype contact with another human person. McGinn and his colleagues say there is potential for robots to do many other more mundane jobs for the elderly, obviating the necessity for a carer who might find little satisfaction in their employment. The pay is often low, and the hours lacking in sociability. In the USA, over 35% of personal carers leave their jobs annually, which is one of the reasons why facilities for the

DOI: 10.4324/9781003186328-6

elderly are often understaffed. There is potential here, however, for freeing up time for carers to have a more meaningful engagement with residents (McGinn, 2017).

For similarly logistic reasons, people living in the community in the UK are regularly tracked by a system known as Technology Integrated Health Management (TIHM), which aims to identify early signs of deterioration of health, to assist people to live for longer in their homes. Some clinical algorithms read the client's physical person for blood pressure, temperature and dehydration signs (Rostill et al., 2019). Even more sophisticated algorithms read the environmental/behavioural data and are able to identify urinary tract infections (UTIs), which are ever-present among people with dementia, especially women. A randomised control trial of the system showed that TIHM identified health issues early on, and therefore reduced the need for hospitalisation among people with dementia (Rostill et al., 2019). This reduction of hospitalisation is a welcome potential outcome, since in older adults who are hospitalised, functional decline can occur in a matter of days (Graf, 2006).

Robots, however, do not necessarily look like people. Moyle et al. (2016; 2018) have researched the use of a robot in the form of a fluffy seal called Paro, using a qualitative approach. Staff in a dementia unit encouraged residents to engage with the seal, and to compare its use as a companion toy to a similar soft animal which was not robotic. The intention behind the research was a reduction in the residents' behavioural and psychological symptoms of dementia. Staff found that the residents engaged more freely with Paro than with the non-automatic look-alike toy. However, findings were mixed, such that the robotic animal should be used differently according to each resident's needs, and not all were comforted by it. Staff also believed the cost of $US6,000 was prohibitive for most aged care facilities.

It is interesting that Moyle et al. (2019) conducted a similar exercise still more recently on the use of life-like non-robotic baby dolls, which have been used throughout aged care services for many years. Their use over time has been ethically controversial for some, verging on the infantilisation of older people with dementia (Mitchell & Templeton, 2014). Researchers used a randomised control trial approach to gauge the likelihood of reducing anxiety, agitation and aggression in the residents. In this investigation, it was clear that the dolls fulfilled the needs of some of the residents and provided pleasure and purposeful activity for them, even though they did not achieve the reduction in symptoms originally aimed for in the research. The learning from these two research projects appears to be that a "one size fits all" approach does not work for this demographic.

Staff shortages in most countries present gaps in the system which are being filled in first world territories by technological benefits for their clients. To keep the regulatory bodies happy, clinicians are expected to spend ever more time on paperwork. Stewart (2011), a visual art therapist, points out that because of this, it is even more significant that arts therapists offer programs designed to meet the goals of the individual clients. It is also recommended that they write up detailed notes and communicate findings while protecting time spent with them (p. 154). She quotes Junge (1994), who says that in the future, we will need to be "particularly nimble contortionists to both continue to be players in the mental arena and yet also retain enough of the freedom which gives spirit and heart to the endeavour of art therapy" (Junge, 1994, p. 281).

With the benefit of hindsight and the rapid expansion of telehealth over almost three decades, Junge's words now seem remarkably prophetic. At the time of writing this chapter in the era of COVID-19, when so many facilities for the aged have fallen prey to infections, the shortage of staff through illness and quarantine has made person-to-person contact even more difficult. This is not helpful when we know that touch is essential for wellbeing (Kitwood, 1997). Governments need to improve systems, rates of pay and training needs for the sector. These essential human needs should be met, and person-centred care (Kitwood, 1997) should still be prioritised and its essential values not bypassed in order to save money. At the 2019 sitting of the Australian Aged Care Royal Commission panel, Daniella Greenwood, a consultant with various aged care facilities, contributed to the view that confusion exists around the nature of technology, and that implementing ideas in aged care doesn't always translate well into good outcomes. Dr Petrovich of Dementia Australia considered that technology as an enabler can serve as an enhancement of quality of life (QoL); however, it should never be offered just because it is available, but for improving QoL for the elderly in general (Royal Commission into Aged Care Quality and Safety, 2019).

Technology for physical and functional care of people with dementia

Before detailing examples of telehealth in the arts therapies, it is important to look at the functional needs of people with dementia at home or in care generally. In the UK, for instance, of the people in residential and nursing homes, 70% now have dementia, an increase from 56% in 2002 (Rostill et al., 2019). Worldwide there are approximately altogether 50 million people affected by dementia (Alzheimer's Disease International, 2020).

An exploratory pilot trial was made into FindMyApps, a program which uses internet-based selection investigated assistance for people with dementia and those who care for them; in this case, appropriate and interesting apps were sourced. This endeavour increased their independence and engagement in enterprising activities (Beentjes et al., 2020). A mixed method investigation was conducted to establish which factors were influencing the initial trial outcomes. The results were uneven, showing that only some of the apps discovered were useful and enjoyable. Some recommendations for changes in the operating systems of tablets used by the cohort were necessitated due to difficulties experienced in the use of touchscreen technology for participants with dementia and their carers.

So far in this book, the case has been made for the essential humanity of life stages in the application of dramatherapy for people with dementia. At the same time, virtual reality (VR) and AI now belong in a range of services for elders who have not grown up with technology. It is true that visual and sound arts technologies and their potential for use in dementia care are constantly being developed to improve their QoL and creative wellbeing. Oliver Sacks (2007) showed with his iPod Project how music through earphones could change the lives of people with Alzheimer's disease. In Australia, the Museum of Contemporary Art (2020) has an online Dementia Toolkit to show people with dementia how to paint (D'Cunha, 2019). Video is an important tool for dramatherapists to offer people so that they can see themselves move and act in the play space; however, real-time confusion can occur for those with dementia and this will be explored in a vignette as part of this chapter. The ethics of using computer technology and AI in therapy will be unpacked, as it addresses (or does not address) the importance of person-centred care at a time when COVID-19 has accelerated and also increased acceptability of the use of technology in aged care and dementia care.

Expressive arts therapy with AI and technology

For older adults without dementia, the Avatar Life Review is a means of employing techniques of more expressive biographical awareness in a hybrid setting of dramatherapy, psychodrama and VR. It explores multiple concepts of self in a "dramatic paradox" and attempts in the process to assist people with mental illnesses, trauma, disabilities and memory loss (Ryu, 2017). Ryu employs the concept of dramatic paradox, explained by dramatherapist Robert Landy (2001), who says that there are manifold sheaths of dramatic experience, naming this as the "dramatic paradox" (2001, p. 380). He believes that because the actor is separate from the role, yet simultaneously merged with it in a coming together of "fictional and non-fictional reality" (1996, p. 11), they exist in a dramatic paradox. A complex and often contradictory set of roles are used here, with the paradox showing itself in the "simultaneous existence of opposites" (Ryu, p. 123) where an avatar of choice is shown on a screen in a theatre environment and the older adult turns to face it. They choose their own avatar out of a selection of eight and are offered the opportunity to play different developmental roles: child, teenager, younger or older adult. This permits the person to take on the role and observe their own performance at the same time as having the dual role of storyteller and listener. Creativity, emerging from the paradox in Ryu's intervention, assists the protagonist to become a more spontaneous story-teller than before.

Writing about the performance cohort, Ryu does not identify the ages or any diagnoses participants may have had, except for mentioning memory loss. She says they possess "the mature psyche of the older adults support(ing) a dual level of consciousness between the lived body and the biological body and between the ageless body and the ageing body" (Faircloth, 2003, p. 81). Since I have been unable to unearth any instances where this type of intervention has been used with people with dementia, I have questions about it as an offering to such people, since it might have the potential to confuse or further confuse them. Nevertheless, it certainly recommends itself for older adults generally, and has the potential to assist them with traumatic memories and mental health issues.

Working with virtual reality during COVID-19

Maxine Radus, a colleague who heads up a creative arts therapy team in a local group of several residential care facilities in Sydney, reports to me that the novelty of working with VR has been welcomed by the elderly residents during a difficult period. She tells me that over the past year, most of the team have felt the weight of restrictions placed on everyday events we take for granted, such as outings. Even under normal circumstances, this is the reality for many living in aged care and makes the use of VR such an attractive prospect. These devices enable them to provide immersive escapism for their clients and interact with virtual replications of both real and unrealistic activities.

Radus advises that the most successful experiences have involved observing/exploring through VR a natural landscape environment, or 360-degree videos of orchestras and circuses. They have trialled the experience of hearing poetry in a setting where the therapist uses a headset along with the person who is seated and have noted that this is the most interactive way to make use of the devices. Optimum results are achieved for the clients when the environment supports the engagement, and when noise is limited to support immersive experience. This type of device has only been used in one-on-one sessions.

There have been some setbacks involved in the new experiences for both staff and clients. Most VR is designed for a much younger target audience. Slower reaction time, poorer vision and reduced balance can turn a game with an appropriate concept or mechanism into a frustrating experience. Lack of experience using handheld controllers and reduced capacity to filter the visual noise that makes up much of the graphical presentation are also barriers to entry. Given that VR technology is quite new, this reduces an already limited number of opportunities to engage in. However, there remains good potential for experiences to be tailored specifically for an aged care setting. Ideally, simpler and "less busy" graphical presentations would be useful, as well as the ability to scale down difficulty levels (e.g. targets are slower or more spaced apart). For this reason, most of their sessions have been experiential with limited direct interaction, as in the nature landscapes already mentioned.

VR for people with dementia: Questions of suitability

Regarding dementia specifically, Radus reports that additional care is required. As VR often aims to completely replace the user's orientation within their surroundings, this poses a risk of confusion. Therapist assessment of the effect and comprehension of the experience is difficult. Discomfort can be further exacerbated for the client by the physical sensation of wearing a headset. Both additional pre-screening for suitability and a therapist with a good understanding of each user's particular presentation of dementia are critical for a beneficial experience for the client.

Telehealth: How does this fit with the needs of people with dementia?

In order to explore the efficacy and appropriateness of dramatherapy with people with dementia in telehealth, it is significant to lay some of the groundwork concerning a trusting human relationship between the therapist and the client. If the therapy has any chance of healing injurious past experiences such as those presented in the pages of this book, it is as important for the therapist to bear in mind questions of attachment and how it influences the relationship, whether the elderly person has dementia or not. Particularly in the case of a person with dementia, it is essential to include the concept of person-centred care and attachment (Kitwood, 1997) in any discussion of some of the separation anxiety and relationship dysfunction that can occur. Strongly connected to this is the question of the use of technology and telehealth with the client, and the required thinking behind their application in dramatherapy. Bowlby described attachment theory as:

> a way of conceptualizing the propensity of human beings to make strong affectional bonds to particular others and of explaining the many forms of emotional distress and personality disturbance, including anxiety, anger, depression, and emotional detachment, to which unwilling separation and loss give rise.
>
> (Bowlby, 1979, p. 127)

In a literature review of attachment theory, ageing and dementia, Browne and Shlosberg (2006) point out that attachment is a significant area of human relationships throughout all stages of a person's life. They show that their research identifies that safe and flourishing attachments at every point in the cycle act as protective factors for later life stages. The quality of the attachment has a bearing on the subjective nature of thoughts and feelings for people with dementia, where estrangement and severance of family bonds tend to be prevailing motifs in dementia care. Despite small samples in the investigations they cover, the authors consider that attachment theory can be a key to finding out why someone with dementia could be displaying particular behaviours. Taking this approach contributes to the design of interventions which are more individual and person-centred (Browne & Shlosberg, 2006).

Examples of early relational experience inducing participant sadness have already been mentioned in Chapter 3, such as Leanne's parents being poor and living "hand to mouth" (Chapter 3, p. 36) and Neil having unfinished business with his father after he died (Chapter 3, p. 37). Informed by the feeling intelligence discussed in the previous chapter (5), the method of defining the self in dementia is inadequate, as it often uses a "purely cognitive method in sociology" (Francis et al., 2020, p. 155). Although poor early attachment may take many forms and is not always an explanation for later problems, its significance in dementia care has often been overlooked (Guthrie & Blood, 2018).

Ethical considerations

In 2015, seven workers were allocated for every elderly person globally, but this is projected to fall to fewer than five in 15 years (United Nations, 2015). This has meant that the research investigating AI for socially assistive robots (SARs) has increased exponentially. These are robots configured to undertake a complicated staged array of activities and tasks designed to convince a client-user that the AI is an interpersonal co-instigator of social interaction (Hegel et al., 2009). When considering the ethics of AI, it is important to remember that robot adoption rates are, however, still very low in the area of dementia (Ienca et al., 2018). In future aged care, however, including care of those with dementia, it is likely AI use will be more viable because of the high cost of caring for people in residential facilities (Alzheimer's Association, 2016). It goes without saying that robot use in aged care precludes much of the possibility of human-to-human contact, which I would argue is almost as destructive in terms of human relational experience as having a robot look after an infant.

Ienca et al. (2018) have reviewed the entire field of intelligence assistive technologies (IATs) for possible use in the future, excluding robots and distinguishing IATs from merely mechanical implements such as conventional walking sticks. The range of IATs includes an array of appliances and systems such as tablets and global positioning system (GPS) trackers: for example; aids for moving around such as electronically powered wheelchairs and walking canes; distributed systems (e.g. sensor systems within the home, mobile platforms, etc.); wearable tracking devices (e.g. for fitness assessment), brain-computer interfaces (BCIs), and software applications for mobile or internet websites (Ienca et al., 2018). The outcome of their investigation of IATs shows that the potential number used for dementia is expanding, with an increase of 400% over five years. As for the technological type, the most common IATs in dementia care are Ambient Assisted Living (AALs) technologies, followed by humanoid robots and handheld devices (Ienca et al., 2018).

The IATs are used not just for clinical purposes, but their application affects the user's feeling and psychosocial life and their relationships with others as well. In 2015, Novitsky et al. comprehensively reviewed the ethics of active assisted living (AAL) technical applications in cases where people have dementia. The relevant issues they found were:

- Users need to have agency in the design and development of these technologies
- There should be informed consent on the part of users
- Social isolation should be considered
- Data security is an ethical issue

Zwijsen et al. (2011) reviewed literature on this topic, looking at the ethical implications of using assisted technologies (ATs) with people in aged care communities, including those with dementia. Agency, freedom and privacy were three ethically meaningful values of concern for stakeholders. There is also a problematic situation where there is inadequate knowledge translation regarding ethical matters in this area. Ethical concerns are seen to be an important barrier to adoption of ATs (Ienca et al., 2018). Boise et al. (2013) have shown in their research on computer monitoring that 60% of participants with mild cognitive impairment had ethical issues connected with privacy and security.

In Malchiodi's (2018) otherwise valuable edited book on art therapy and digital technology, there is only one reference to dementia connected with technology, and that is in an art therapy assessment aligned with a clinical assessment of severity of dementia. The participants are asked to fill out mandala templates manually, and the colours and patterns of drawing are assessed by a computer statistical regression method (Seong-In, 2018). It seems logical to draw the conclusion that for Malchiodi and her contributors, technology in art therapy with this cohort of people was not their area of interest.

When working with people in a life stage and situation where interpersonal connection is such a valuable relational asset in being human, it is certainly important to think carefully about which technologies are appropriate. Interaction on Zoom could be confusing for people with dementia. In an experience with a group of people in residential care or at a day centre, a wholly intersubjective space where people could interact in a circle is rec-ommended, rather than in small rectangles on Zoom. The following pro-ject certainly used technology to create a film; however, the dramatherapist offering the program for it needed the clients to be face to face.

A vignette of a film-making project highlighting the stories of people with dementia

In 2019, Dannielle Jackson, a dramatherapist, ran a programme called "Drama Connections" at three different facilities under the rubric of Integrated Living Aged Care Centres on the Central Coast of New South Wales. The work was facilitated in ten-week segments, time-sharing between three of their activity centres there. Offering various dramather-apy interventions and techniques, the clients worked with their individual stories to build interpersonal trust and get to know each other. They also explored and took roles in fairy tales and fables to bring humour and play into the programme, while developing their performance skills. Dress-ups and props were often used to accompany the stories and these provided clients with the opportunity to be spontaneous in their creativity. These initial sessions were the first steps in bringing together the three groups on film, culminating in a collaboration that resulted in ensemble work, and then became a short film (Cheu, 2019). The film was a great success and was the winner in the section "Best memory support programme to engage, enable rehabilitation and happiness for older adults with demen-tia" at the World Ageing Festival (2020) in Singapore. The category in the Asia Pacific Elder Care Innovation Awards was "Best Dementia Care Programme".

In the following vignette, Jackson presents her narrative of the rationale for the program and the way her facilitation allowed the client-led aspects of the project to unfold. Names have been changed to protect confidentiality.

> When I first met George, he wanted to leave the centre because he didn't feel he belonged there. We slowly started writing short poems based on what we called 'life photographs'. As George's trust and familiarity developed, so too did the poems, to include movement and dialogue. George suggested that he wanted to share what we were creating with his wife, so we decided to film it with an appropriate set, costumes, props and background music. This was arranged for one of his poems, which was about an encounter where he escaped a bush fire by hiding under a water trough. It resulted in loud laughter from onlookers who were amazed that he was able to walk away unharmed, while George's wife was moved to tears. I realised that there was also potential through the witnessing of a client's dramatherapy engagement to provide signif-icant comfort for their loved ones.

Planning began on an ambitious idea involving three separate centres, each with 15 clients, to create one 'cinema quality' film based on meaningful personal content. Considerations were made regarding client suitability accompanied by participant interviews to set personal goals. For safety reasons, given the neurocognitively disparate range of clients with whom I was simultaneously working, the sessions focused on exploring strengths-based stories of personal achievements, contributions and moments of personal significance in one's life. However, in the interest of remaining client-focused and in anticipation of deeper content arising in the group, a flexible hour was allocated at the end of each group session to spend with any client one on one who needed further support.

Group sessions began with a story that explored a loose theme each week such as love, change, loss and desire (themes determined by what arose in the previous session). Clients were prompted with sensory materials to share lived experiences surrounding each topic. Some of these moments became titles for developing imaginary stories, while others were played out, always accompanied by another client (or myself) playing narrator so as not to confuse any clients during the role plays. Whilst exploring envy, Betty shared a memory about her neighbours' kids who would steal apricots from her tree. One day, out of frustration, she made a large batch of apricot jam for them all to share. The group role-played eating the delicious homemade jam while Betty, also in role, beamed with pride.

After eight weeks we had a large collection of stories in which everyone had contributed at least one personal memory. I approached Brian - a former journalist living with moderate Alzheimer's - to work with me and assist in the impossible task of incorporating the stories into a single narrative script. He immediately pulled out a pen and pad from his top pocket and started taking notes. Then came art making/building sets and costumes which included collaborations with other creative therapists.

I jump forward to the film day. This looked like the scene of any professional film set complete with camera crew, lighting, sound equipment, even a makeup station. Some clients did feel overwhelmed with the activity, were nervous or confused and were not therefore able to play roles on the day. These people could take on other duties to stay connected with the group such as dressing the set, taking the clapper role, calling 'Action', holding the boom, or at the very least had a front row seat to witness it all.

When I had first met Catherine, she had been wary of other clients. She would hide her face inside her jumper, verbally abuse people as they walked past or on occasion throw her coffee and food. Through role identification she was able to express that she felt like an angry person;

during session she was given a safe opportunity to stand in front of the group to be an angry person. Once the anger was released her mood turned quickly to laughter. I mention Catherine since a major consideration of any therapeutic practice is to meet the client where they are at any given day. Catherine used her temperament in the film by playing a security guard who found everyone else frustrating; she would shake her head or make hand gestures of dismissal. By granting her permission to be expressive in this way her anger turned to humour and she appeared to find the whole process very amusing.

The day finally came for people from the three centres to meet for the first time and watch their work on the big screen. My first days in the centres had been met with shyness, sometimes disinterest or avoidance, but now they came together to watch themselves be stars on a large cinema screen. More importantly they had an opportunity to be more than their condition, more than their limitations; their loved ones, staff and the organisation were able to share that enjoyment too. I recall a shared sense of pride and achievement among the participants:

- Brian asked if we could write a sequel
- Betty was excited to tell me that SHE was in a movie
- Catherine gave me a hug and the biggest smile I had ever seen on her face
- George told me at the screening, the therapy reminded him he's not an idiot

However, it should be mentioned that although the technical elements of the project were necessary and celebrated by the clients, this could not have been achieved in any way except face to face in preparation for the final filming. Ultimately the process was a success due to two factors; firstly a well-established 'in person' group that supported and trusted one another after a series of weeks together, and secondly their moderate (not severe) stage in decline.

(As a registered dramatherapist, facilitator and therapeutic programmer, Dannielle Jackson works with dementia, disability, families experiencing domestic violence and at-risk youth. Her practice is born from her professional theatre background and influenced by Rudolf Steiner as well as Indigenous Australian stories.)

Finally, having explored some of the available benefits of AI and technology in this chapter, it seems appropriate to submit an example of a face-to-face session with my research cohort which would have been impossible to offer to people with dementia by means of either of these alternatives. This session shows how immediate and powerful face-to-face work can be in encouraging interpersonal connection. My reason for including this sessional work in a chapter on technology is to illustrate how important it is to have people face to face in the same room to do the work of dramatherapy. Like Jackson's cohorts, trust between group members had built up over eight weeks, and they were far more relaxed with me and one another than they had been at the start of the program. On a normal Zoom gathering, they would not be able to work in partnership, and even in breakout rooms, they would be more self-conscious and missing out on the combined energy of the animal conversation.

Session 8: Celebrating ourselves

The session was the last of our weekly sessions before a break of two weeks. It had been preceded by a session on grief, which was a mini preparation for the final ending of the program in 11 weeks' time. The group gathered and talked about a very competitive football game between Queensland and New South Wales, and then there were a few reflections on the previous week's work. A few warm-up games were played, including Pass the Balloon, Cat and Mouse and then Grandmother's/Grandfather's Footsteps (see Appendix Session 8 for references). There was an intentional rationale for so many warm-ups; I had observed a video of a particular activity – Cat and Dog – by David Howe at the British Association of Dramatherapists Conference in 2010, and I wanted to offer it in this celebratory session. Each participant chose a partner and chose who would take the role of a cat and who a dog. I instructed them not to use the language of humans, but only to use animal sounds, giving them a brief demonstration of both types of sounds. They then proceeded to have paired conversations in cat and dog language.

The result was nothing short of astonishing. Even those who regularly were shy or unwilling to take part in warm-ups entered into it with great gusto. The animal sounds were varied – some loud and some soft, and some took on the body language of the animal they were improvising. There were sounds of disappointment when I first asked them to swap roles, so I gave them a little more time before the changeover. When the conversations finally came to an end, they reflected with enthusiasm with their partners on how this had been for them. The work in dyads had freed them from any anxiety about retrieving words, thanks to the example of communication in the animal kingdom. In the following session entitled Animal kingdom, participants modelled the animals they had improvised (see the figurine of the dog in Figure 6.1).

This warm-up was followed by an extremely enthusiastic enactment of Magic Box (Johnson, 1986; Sandel & Johnson, 1987), an intervention which is explained in Chapter 3, pp. 34–35. The spontaneous activity was interesting, especially for a last session when participants knew they would have a break before returning to group sessions. There were conversations about depression and whether it goes up or down and an improvised celebratory

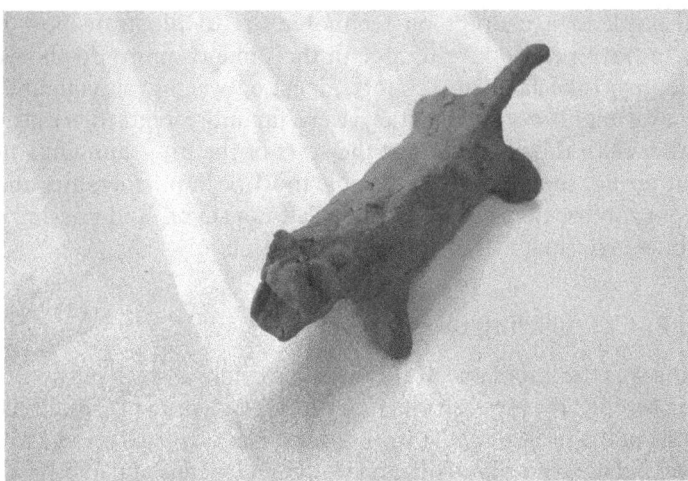

Figure 6.1 Clay dog

meal in a restaurant, all culminating in a worship of Paul, one of the group elders, who "en-roled" as an ancient Roman statue. (Paul had been an architect who took groups of interested tourists around Italy's monuments and galleries in his retirement.) Each of the other participants laid down a coloured cloth at his feet in tribute, which appeared to symbolise a ritual celebration of Paul as the elder and main source of wisdom of the group. (These improvisations will be discussed more fully in Chapter 8.) This ritualised show of respect for a treasured elder was both a fitting and moving way to end, before participants sang the final song: "Every time we say goodbye" (Porter, 1981).

References

Alzheimer's Association. (2016). 2016 Alzheimer's disease facts and figures. *Alzheimer's & Dementia*, *12*(4), 459–509.

Alzheimer's Disease International. (2020). *About dementia*. Retrieved November 12, 2020, from https://www.alz.co.uk/about-dementia

Beentjes, J. M., Kerkhof, Y. J. F., Neal, D. P., Teake, P., Koppelle, M. A., Meiland, F. J. M., Graff, M., & Moes, R.-M. (2020). Process evaluation of the FindMyApps program trial of people with dementia or MCI and their caregivers based on the MCR guidance. *Gerontechnology*, *20*(5), 1–15.

Boise, L., Wild, K., Mattek, N., Ruhl, M., Dodge, H. H., & Kaye, J. (2013). Willingness of older adults to share data and privacy concerns after exposure to unobtrusive in-home monitoring. *Gerontechnology: International Journal on the Fundamental Aspects of Technology to Serve the Ageing Society*, *11*(3), 428–435.

Bowlby, J. (1979). *The making and breaking of affectional bonds*. Tavistock.

Browne, C. J., & Shlosberg, E. (2006). Attachment theory, ageing and dementia: A review of the literature. *Aging and Mental Health, 10*(2), 134–142.

Cheu, S. (2019). Australian ageing agenda. Retrieved December 3, 2020, from www.Australianageingagenda.com.au

D'Cunha, N. (2019). *Getting to the "art" of dementia.* University of Canberra. Retrieved November 18, 2019, from https://www.canberra.edu.au/uncover/news-archive/2019/november/getting-to-the-art-of-dementia-new-research-highlights-benefits-of-art-intervention

Faircloth, C. (2003). *Aging bodies: Images & everyday experience.* Altamira Press.

Francis, L. E., Lively, K. J., Konig, A., & Hoey, J. (2020). The affective self: Perseverance of self-sentiments in late-life dementia. *Social Psychology Quarterly, 83*(2), 153–172.

Graf, C. L. (2006). Functional decline in older adults: It's often a consequence of hospitalisation, but it doesn't have to be. *The American Journal of Nursing, 106*(1), 58–67.

Guthrie, L., & Blood, I. (2018). *Supporting older people using attachment-informed and strength-based approaches.* Jessica Kingsley.

Hegel, F., Muhl, C., Wrede, B., Hielscher-Fastabend, M., & Sagerer, G. (2009). Understanding social robots. *Second International Conference of Advanced Computer Interaction Section II*: 169–174. https://aiweb.techfak.uni-bielefeld.de/files/2009%20hegel%20ACHI.pdf

Howe, D. (2010). Forget-me-not: How dramatherapy meets the theatre of everyday life in dementia care settings. *Presentation at Annual Conference of The British Association of Dramatherapists*, Durham University, UK.

Ienca, M., Wangmo, T., Jotterand, F., Kressig, R. W., & Elger, B. (2018). Ethical design of intelligent assistive technologies for dementia: A descriptive review. *Scientific Engineering Ethics, 24*, 1035–1055.

Johnson, D. (1986). The developmental method in dramatherapy: Group treatment with the elderly. *The Arts in Psychotherapy, 13*, 17–33.

Junge, M. B. (with Asawa, P.). (1994). A history of art therapy in the United States. *American Art Therapy Association, 11*(3), 175–179.

Kitwood, T. (1997). *Dementia reconsidered.* Open University Press.

Landy, R. (1996). *Persona and performance: The meaning of role in drama, therapy, and everyday life.* The Guilford Press.

Landy, R. (2001). *New essays in drama therapy.* Charles C. Thomas.

Malchiodi, C. (2018). *The handbook of art therapy and digital technology.* Jessica Kingsley.

McGinn, C. (2017, November). We built a robot – care assistant for elderly people: Here's how it works. *The Conversation.* https://theconversation.com/we-built-a-robot-care-assistant-for-elderly-people-heres-how-it-works-87108

Mitchell, G., & Templeton, M. (2014). Ethical considerations of doll therapy for people with dementia. *Nursing Ethics, 21*(6), 720–730.

Moyle, W., Bramble, M., Jones, C., & Murfield, J. (2018). Care staff perceptions of a social robot called Paro and a look-alike plush toy: A descriptive, qualitative approach. *Aging and Mental Health, 22*(3), 330–335.

Moyle, W., Jones, C., Sung, B., Bramble, M., O'Dwyer, S., Blumenstein, M., & Estivill-Castro, V. (2016). What effect does an animal robot called Cuddler have on the engagement and emotional response of older people with dementia? A pilot feasibility study. *International Journal of Social Robotics, 8*, 145–156.

Moyle, W., Murfield, J., Jones, C., Beattie, E., Draper, B., & Ownsworth, T. (2019). Can life-like baby dolls reduce symptoms of anxiety, agitation or aggression for people with dementia in long-term care? Findings from a pilot randomised control trial. *Aging & Mental Health*, *23*(10), 1442–1450.

Museum of Contemporary Art. (2020) *Artful program for people with dementia*. Retrieved August 30, 2020, from https://www.mca.com.au/learn/art-dementia

Porter, C. (1981). *Every time we say goodbye*. Chappell & Co., Inc.

Rostill, H., Nilforooshan, R., Morgan, A., Barnaghi, P., Ream, E., & Chrysanthaki, T. (2019). Technology integrated health management for dementia. *British Journal of Community Nursing*, *23*(10), 502–508.

Royal Commission into Aged Care Quality and Safety. (2019). Retrieved from https://agedcare.royalcommission.gov.au/publications/interim-report

Ryu, S. (2017). Avatar life-review: Virtual bodies in a dramatic paradox. *Virtual Creativity*, *7*(2), 121–131.

Sacks, O. (2007). *Musicophilia*. Vintage Books.

Sandel, S., & Johnson, D. (1987). *Waiting at the gate: Creativity & hope in the nursing home*. The Haworth Press.

Seong-In, K. (2018). Computational art therapy in art therapy assessment and research. In C. Malchiodi (Ed.), *The handbook of art therapy and digital technology* (pp. 348–372). Jessica Kingsley.

Stewart, E. G. (2011). Art therapy and neuroscience blend: Working with people who have dementia. *Art Therapy: Journal of the American Art Therapy Association*, *21*(3), 148–155.

United Nations. (2015). *United Nations world population prospects*. http://esa.un.org/unpd/wpp/Publications/Files/WPP2015_Volume-I_Comprehensive-Tables.Pdf

World Ageing Festival. (2020). *8th Asia-Pacific Eldercare Innovation Awards: Winner*. Retrieved December 3, 2020, from https://worldageingfestival.heysummit.com/8th-asia-pacific-eldercare-innovation-awards/

Zwijsen, S. A., Niemeijer, A. R., & Hertogh, C. M. P. M. (2011). Ethics of using assistive technology in the care for community-dwelling elderly people: An overview of the literature. *Aging Mental Health*, *15*(4), 419–427.

Chapter 7

Trauma and intersubjectivity in dementia

This chapter explores trauma-informed dramatherapy, with particular reference to the artistic application of methods and techniques which have helped to give elders permission to deal with difficult memories regarding complex trauma. It follows a chapter which documents the proliferation of artificial intelligence (AI) yet encourages interpersonal human connection. The chapter aims to present additional reasons why such connection is important, due to the frequent presence of unaddressed trauma response in people with dementia.

Responses to childhood trauma are considered along with their effects and the need for these to be addressed early on in life. These factors may be separate from the onset of trauma responses later in life which may occur as a result of war and other major events, sometimes of a social nature. Connected with trauma response, the diagnosis of post-traumatic stress disorder (PTSD) is defined and considered. In the recent past, studies have explored the possibility that trauma in childhood or middle age may be two of many factors which affect the onset of dementia later in life. Other unrelated and more widely known physical factors are considered here also. Session plans are referred to and provided as guides to the health professional working with people with dementia. Vignettes illustrate the interpersonal nature of trauma as experienced through dramatherapy and how this was experienced and expressed in sessions.

What are some of the known causes of the onset of dementia?

Dementia Australia (2021) tells us that some of the causes are still unknown, and we are still learning about them. We do know, however, that there are gene mutations which can be directly responsible for the onset of Alzheimer's disease (AD) and some other dementias. There are beta-amyloid plaque deposits and neuro-fibrillary tangles in the brain (mentioned in Chapter 2) which are more common in people with AD and some other forms of dementia (Dementia Australia, 2021). These are not always present

DOI: 10.4324/9781003186328-7

at autopsy in someone with dementia as Snowden (2001), when investigating the autopsy evidence of older women for his Nun Study, clearly showed. His research was done before the availability of tomography such as CAT or MRI, which now show absence or presence clearly in the living person.

Vascular Dementia can be caused by high blood pressure, small strokes and abnormal patterns of heartbeat which cause blockages in the blood vessels. Autoimmune arterial diseases such as lupus can also exacerbate the blockages; in Binswanger's disease, the brain's nerve fibres can also affect blood flow, causing Vascular Dementia.

Lewy Bodies Dementia is caused by small, round entities which lodge in and affect the nerve cells in the brain. This dementia type can co-occur with the previous two types and investigations have not ascertained why the Lewy bodies appear. Other causes of dementia have been found to be the Kreutzfeld-Jakob type, which is rare and is otherwise known as "mad cow disease", and also the Huntington type, which is caused by an inherited mutation of the gene of the same name. Over-indulgence in alcohol can also be a causative factor for dementia (Dementia Australia, 2021).

Post-traumatic stress disorder

In World War II (WWII), PTSD was still little understood, even though occasional treatments were recommended for what was known as "soldiers' heart" in the American Civil War and as "shell shock" in World War I victims (Butterworth, 2018). Gradually, the symptoms of trauma experienced by those who fought in or experienced the tragedy of World War II began to be recognised as serious symptoms of traumatic memories of what they had seen and done in wartime. However, more women are raped each year than soldiers killed or traumatised in battle. PTSD was recognised in women long after it had been recognised in veterans. The extent of wartime rape is shocking in its proportions, although actual numbers are very difficult to come by (Lamb, 2020). PTSD has since been applied to trauma experienced much earlier in life as well, so these combined facts tell us that PTSD is more common than we might believe. It is usually a cluster of stress responses that can ensue as a result of experiencing violent physical or sexual behaviour, a death or an accident, or witnessing a traumatic occurrence happen to someone else (Black Dog Institute, 2021).

Symptoms associated with this disorder, especially for war veterans, are: an intense experience of living through the event (see Tanya's and Leanne's experiences in the vignettes below), avoiding reminders of it, jumping at loud noises, negative changes in beliefs, negative feelings and thoughts about it and feeling on edge or unable to sleep, sometimes because of nightmares. Other common symptoms for people experiencing PTSD include recurrent memories of the event, apathy and a lack of interest, numbness to feeling, outbursts of anger, or being constantly on guard (hyperarousal). High blood pressure can result, with the body experiencing sweating or blushing, with elevated levels of cortisol caused by fear in the pit of the stomach. Disengagement and disassociation can also occur. The DSM-5 (American Psychiatric Association, 2013) and the ICD-11 (ICD-11, 2019) have slightly different criteria for PTSD. The latter favours a more complex set of symptomatic elements and a wider diagnosis intended to include the ongoing intrusive thoughts that can be brought about by exposure to trauma and are sometimes dismissed as hallucinations.

According to several neuroscientists, there is evidence of a reduction in the volume and connectivity of the hippocampus with some forms of dementia and with ageing (as they argue to be the case in AD [Allen et al., 2007]). This is thought to be connected to cognitive deficits associated with PTSD (Vasterling et al., 2002, as cited in Yehuda & LeDoux, 2007). The depleted hippocampus could cause problems with the process whereby people's reaction to trauma is put into context and integrated in a thoughtful pathway that could lead to a recovery response. In this case, limitations to cognitive resilience could handicap recovery (Yehuda & LeDoux, 2007). They recommend taking note of the most elementary neuroscience research which can help to predict the need for investigation when viewed through a developmental lens. Changes reflecting a high degree of PTSD and ageing, diverging from the commonly regarded patterns of PTSD or elderhood regarding cortisol and hippocampal changes, can be detected in MRI tomography. This knowledge can present greater understanding of risk, levels of PTSD, and the presence of chronic results of trauma response, because it takes into account the life stage of the person experiencing trauma. There may also be hyperarousal in the amygdala, which can be responsible for chronic hypervigilance and a fear response, as well as the disassociation that can be seen in responses like some of Tanya's and Ben's in the vignettes below.

There are major events which are still having an impact now on people of an age to be diagnosed with dementia. These people are living longer than used to be the case, due to the improvements in hygiene and higher standard of living today. Their age range is from approximately 70 years old to 100. In the USA, from a total of 142,246 veterans who had been prisoners of war serving in Korea, Vietnam and in World War II, almost 30,000 were still alive at the end of 2005 (Klein et al., quoted in Meziab et al., 2014). Yaffe et al. (2010) reported that veterans returning from the Vietnam War had a 20% to 30% prevalence of experience of PTSD lasting a lifetime, and 10–15% were suffering from this condition 15 years or more after returning from Vietnam. A study of older veterans of World War II and the Korean war found they were 12% more likely than others to experience PTSD symptoms after the war had been over for 45 years (quoted in Yaffe et al., 2010). Yaffe and her co-researchers wanted to find out whether PTSD is responsible for the possibility of later onset of dementia in a mixed gender but mainly male cohort of older veterans of the US armed services who were being treated in the official veterans' medical clinics. They found that those with PTSD were at a two-fold higher risk of developing dementia after their return than those who had no PTSD (Yaffe et al., 2010). In 2018, Barnes et al. came to a similar conclusion regarding veterans of the Iraq and Afghanistan wars who had mild traumatic brain injury (MTBI) without loss of consciousness, and risk was over two-fold higher than those with no MTBI (Barnes, et al., 2018). Thus, both the psychological and physical dangers of war have had far-reaching effects, increasing the risk of dementia.

Groups of older people who have suffered from PTSD in connection with civil wars and living in other war zones are the many ethnically diverse people who have needed to flee their countries, such as Syrians, Iraqis, Afghanis and many more, perhaps because of war, but also because of persecution and civil war in their own regions. Dislocation issues and experiences of torture or dangerous sea crossings in small boats can intensify the symptoms of PTSD. The resulting behaviour of older people experiencing these issues linked to immigration can cause health professionals to mistake the memories of torture and trauma for behavioural and psychological symptoms of dementia (BPSD). It is therefore essential that the history of these individuals be researched as thoroughly as possible, and it is not always easy to do this because of language difficulties. Memory flashes from the past can be misconstrued as hallucinations (the latter being possible symptoms of dementia), hypervigilance as a neurotic disorder and hyperactivity as perseverance. How often has an elderly person been restrained in a nursing home which is short-staffed or has unethical systems, when aggressive behaviour results? Rather than "bad behaviour", this response could easily be a trauma reaction to imprisonment or even torture.

Other research has established causal links between trauma, PTSD and dementia unrelated to war experience, with PTSD being a possible cause of dementia (Craftman et al., 2020; Flannery, 2002). Further reasons for unaddressed trauma are epidemics like the Ebola virus or the polio epidemics. Polio affected many countries in the world after World War II, causing health shocks and paralysis to young children and adolescents. Findings from research on the version that occurred in Denmark in 1952 (Gensowski et al., 2019) show that childhood disability from polio increased the likelihood of early retirement and disability pension receipt at age 50, and although there was no significant difference between people with and without ongoing paralysis, the risk of early death for patients with paralysis was higher for children from low socio-economic groups than those from more advantaged circumstances.

Does childhood trauma affect later onset of dementia?

It is possible that a misinterpretation of the aetiology of dementia combined with mixing its classifications has exceeded the limits of the term "dementia" (Hachinski, 2008). According to Kivipelto and Solomon (2009), understanding of the term should move from this category and the question could be asked: "quel est le risque de developer une démence en vieillissant, en lien avec une enfance traumatique?" (Clément, 2012). In other words, she questions the risk of developing dementia, in later life, linked to a traumatic childhood.

Clément argues that there are many factors early in life which can contribute to complex traumatic responses, such as lack of education, poverty and lack of opportunity, as in the Danish study above, quite apart from physical, sexual or emotional abuse. Obviously, there are also protective factors during a long life, but these may not be enough to repair damage. Cook and Simiola (2018) argue that trauma is "less well-researched, under-recognised and under-treated in older as opposed to younger populations" (p. 7). They find scarce interest in referring such people for psychotherapy to deal with their PTSD.

Yukako Tani et al. (2020) investigated the links between difficult experiences when young and a diagnosis of dementia among Japanese people born before 1948. She and her team assessed 17,412 individuals taken from the Japan Gerontological Evaluation Study, a census investigation of people 65 years and older. Seven childhood adverse and traumatic experiences were assessed: parental death, parental divorce, parental mental illness, family violence, physical abuse, psychological neglect, and psychological abuse. Using Cox regression measures, it was found that an incidence of three or more such experiences was linked to an increased threat of being diagnosed with dementia as an adult.

It is a sad fact that this research is only just now bearing fruit and that families and carers in residential and nursing homes are not yet aware of it. There are instances of people with dementia in care whose families report that their first presentation for diagnosis is how they have always been. Gerrard (2019) writes about a woman in the dementia section of a large hospital trust in the UK who was endlessly calling out and visibly upset. The nursing staff, who believed in their patients' basic humanity, however erratic and confused they were, saw them as people who are meaningful and in possession of a self. They told the family this was not normal to be constantly distraught and that the woman was informing them of something significant. They discovered that she had long suffered from unchecked arthritis, which was why she was so distressed, and they were able to help her with it. Or the woman whose husband had never seen her without clothes, even though they had three children and no one else had seen her naked either. No wonder she refused a shower (Gerrard, 2019). Trauma can come in various terrible disguises and neglect is not always given the same weight as violent abuse, but it is still abuse.

Inter-generational trauma is rarely mentioned in the literature on dementia, but this experience can be applied to older adults who have collectively faced historical traumas, such as Indigenous people. Many people with an Australian aboriginal background were removed from their parents as children and are now experiencing dementia (Radford et al., 2017) and Indigenous people are more generally three times more likely to experience dementia than is the case in other Australian population groups. Dementia occurs at younger ages in relation to other demographics, AD being the more usual diagnosis (Radford et al., 2015; Smith et al., 2008, as cited in Radford et al., 2017). Ageing Holocaust survivors as well as LGBTQ older adults are also extremely vulnerable (Stern & Hulko, 2016). Craftman et al. (2020) in an ethical enquiry into Holocaust survivors with dementia, found that nursing care "needed to be based on both in-depth, contemporary knowledge of the trauma (here WWII) and the individual's life story" (p. 630). Neuroscientists tell us that the neurocognitive deficits in ageing survivors of such traumatic events, and responses such as intrusive memories, processing thoughts, somatic and emotional changes, add to people's distress and make them more vulnerable in response to treatment (Rehman et al., 2020).

Complex trauma in the arts therapies

More than 30 years ago, arts therapists were working with clients experiencing trauma and with PTSD (Read Johnson, 1987). Herman (1992) warned early on that a specialised approach was needed to assist people suffering the impact of violent assault and abuse. Response to complex trauma is usually interpersonal, often recurrent, and includes feeling cornered or ambushed in some way, including by the overwhelm of deep feelings of shame and loss of identity in managing traumatic emotions (Blue Knot Foundation, 2019).

World Health Organization global researchers have found that survivors of violent abuse carry the highest PTSD lifetime burden of risk for respondents across surveys in countries where average incomes are median or low (Kessler et al., 2018, p. 12). Interpersonal violence is a global challenge and has serious long-term impacts on every level (Sethi & Butchart, 2017). Arts therapy clients often seek help because of symptoms of PTSD; however, they sometimes arrive at sessions completely unaware of the causes of these signs. Symptoms can include physical indications, such as racing heart, problems with breathing, disassociation, tension in the muscles, or mental symptoms of anxiety (Jaaniste & Perry, 2021).

Neurocognitive symptoms are also found to exacerbate PTSD likelihood as well as leading to an increased risk of developing dementia in later life. Additionally, the witnessing of traumatic events happening to others may induce a traumatic response in the observer. Various approaches to creative and expressive arts therapy, sometimes intermodal, have been offered to people impacted by trauma for some time, with an emphasis on the person-centred relationship as the core principle of all active treatment (Carey, 2006; Webb, 2004). Porges' (1997, 2004) polyvagal theory has contributed to the research for the study of tension, emotion and communal behaviour. His theory provides a link between the evolvement of the autonomic nervous system and emotional experience, perceptual expression, voiced communication and associated social behaviour. Peter Levine (1997) has been influenced by Porges' embodiment work, developing a method he calls "resourcing", assisting clients to be somatically present through breathing, playing or singing. Van der Kolk's (2002) research has revealed that visual memories and those associated with movement gathered in the brain can be positively affected without entering into the trauma narrative (Jaaniste & Perry, 2021). He states that the contribution worldwide of creative arts therapies assisting people with trauma may be "to circumvent the speech-lessness that comes with terror" (van der Kolk, 2014, p. 243).

Other ways to circumvent both the loss of voice and avoidance of traumatic memories are found in the stories we tell ourselves as human beings in order to protect us from the burden of grief. (These stories will be dealt with further in the next chapter on grief and loss in old age.) Nicci Gerrard (2019) records her mother's avoidance story of a memory from childhood before she received the diagnosis of dementia. As a nine-year-old in 1941, her mother was fleeing from Palestine with family. The ship they were escaping in blew up in the Gulf of Suez and they were helped into a lifeboat, watching the ship slowly sink. Her mother would tell the story of being picked up and put into the lifeboat by a robust young man. When they were back in a secure place on land, someone said a handbag had been found – important for those leaving Palestine with all their worldly goods. It turned out to be her mother's precious bag of toys, containing no money or wealth. This was the story she told all her adult life.

In fact, the bombing of the ship had resulted in an oil spill which had caught fire, and the surface of the ocean had been burning. In the water were neighbours and friends of their family, simultaneously burning and drowning, calling out to be rescued. The lifeboats, filled to the gunnels with too many already to take on more, were rowed through the people in the sea and she could recognise their faces in the fire. Her mother's memory of the toy bag had been a protective barrier against this terrible memory until old age and dementia. Gerrard says that in dementia, the ability to hold nuanced balance between memories kept and memories let go of can disappear. She says that the remote past can rush back uninvited with clarity, whether welcomed or not. At the same time, memories that are fresher can fragment and vanish (2019). I include this story in order to emphasise the possibility that what can be seen by care staff or family as "emotive behaviour", impassioned perseverance or inappropriate responses to a situation, can in fact be a real re-emergence of a genuine response to trauma.

Interpersonal response to people with dementia, in addition to treatment

Above all, people with dementia need a warm, human connection. Their chosen name should always be respected, and being addressed as "darling" and "love" can be very patronising. These people should never be talked down to, and can tell very easily if they are being treated like children. It is important to be very clear in conversation, and not to use any jargon. When they are in the earlier stages of dementia, their conversation will be responsive and reasonably clear, but as they lose more words and the skills required to get around word loss, it will be more difficult. They need eye contact and speech that is slow and considered, and good listeners to their stories. If they have the full attention of their speaking partner, it will be much easier for them and for the partner to help with ends of sentences or further questioning to understand their meaning. People need touch, as they are often isolated, so a light pat on the arm can be a great help with verbal flow. Above all, it is important to enter the world of the person. On a good day, they may be right on target with the subject, but on a bad day, they may be living in the past like Gerrard's mother, and the memories may be unspeakably painful. In busy care homes, the hastening advance of the clock can be all-important for staff, but how much warmer to be invited into the dining room for lunch, rather than told to hurry up because it's lunchtime. In a group, it is important to act as a conversational link between one person and another, as when one's world shrinks, it is not always easy to remember that others are present. For people in the final stages of dementia, gesture can be very important for both conversational partners, and if an immigrant has lost words and speaks in their original language, it is good to try and communicate through gesture or find an interpreter if possible. Aggression rarely occurs when the person with dementia has the full attention of the hearer.

Traumatic experiences and responses in the dramatherapy group

The oldest female member of the dramatherapy group, Tanya (88), came into more than one session saying that she had no idea who had brought her from home that day. All she could remember was the day when, at the age of 16, Hitler's troops had marched into her hometown of Vienna in 1938. This was a memory of the trauma of the occupation by the Third Reich when the Jewish people living there were treated with such cruelty and humiliation by the Gestapo and others. In Vienna, Eichmann archived all Jewish men as Israel and women as Sara, eliminating their identity. The first shock of seeing those soldiers march in must have been so terrible, especially as she was aware that her father was a Socialist. The re-lived experience of that entire episode in Tanya's life was a post-traumatic stress response.

We had first heard her story in Session 3:

TANYA: You know, to see these Nazis walking down, yelling Heil Hitler and all that sort of stuff and my father who was a social democrat and a left-wing party member and well and truly exposed, you know. And I know he was head of … that was when I was 16, 17 years old.

Tanya told us that after some time, her courageous father had organised with friends to help the family escape to Holland. From there, they came to Australia. I decided on hearing her story in this third session, risky as it was so near the beginning, to ask everyone to get into the now invisible train which had been so scary for her back then, not knowing whether they would get to Holland without being discovered. It was an intentional decision, based on Levine's (1997) theory of resourcing through socialisation and the positive interpersonal responses I was sure she would receive from this interaction. Tanya was a woman who lived alone, with occasional visits from her son. We all improvised rattling along in the train together, and participants groaned occasionally as I provided some narrative that questioned where or how we would get out. She had told us a guard had come around to look at passports, and they had got through that. We just concentrated hard on the destination – Holland.

TANYA: Oh it, it, – but I don't know why it's coming back to me just now.

JOANNA: How do you get out of here?

BEN: I don't know.

NEIL: *(pointing)* There's the door. There's the exit.

TANYA: And the border guard came and … And we did get through.

JOANNA: You did get through. Did you hear that?

TANYA: Well of course.

JOANNA: Ok. Now we're going to be where the train stopped and we're still very worried. Are we going to get out? Everybody, are we going to get out? Are we going to get out?

TANYA: And you know the guards, and then they let us go through.

PAUL: And we're not going to get out might be the *(nervous laughter)*

TANYA: Well, I was 16 years old.

LEANNE: It could be worse.

TANYA: And my mother, who was such a simple woman – anyhow I'm a five months baby, you know. She was pregnant so he married her. But you know, she was a simple woman and she really couldn't understand it. And her family didn't want her to leave and – oh, it was just such a …

JOANNA: You know what we're going to do now? *(The train stopping at the station)*.

TRUDY: Oh God, yes.

JOANNA: Look at – look at what, um, Neil's doing. Hah.

NEIL: Breathe.

Finally, the train had stopped and we piled out. Neil called out to everyone to breathe and people mirrored him as he stretched out his arms, while Tanya exclaimed, "The guards let us through!"

In reflecting on this brief intervention, Tanya talked about the drama of being in that carriage, even in improvised form. It seemed as though the whole group was speaking for her as well as themselves, saying that they were relieved, happy and these positive feelings spilled over into the group. It is upsetting and suffocating for all to be on a journey of dementia, not knowing whether their lives will deteriorate further and this seemed to be the metaphor they were enacting.

When we finally arrived in "Holland" (extending the metaphor: perhaps an oasis from dementia's relentless onset), members of the group expressed feelings of freedom, joy and surprise after de-roling from exposure to risk and anxiety in role.

De-roling "has a function to assist the player to leave the role and return to their normal reality" (Jones, 2007, p. 216). This often means that the dramatherapist encourages the participant to shake their body energetically, de-identifying themselves from the role they have played. They can shake off a childhood pet name and say their present name if they have taken a role from a young life stage. Care must be taken to make sure that everyone is de-roled once a performance has taken place.

Exposing people to difficult memories attempts to help clients to be less sensitive to elements associated with the trauma. Such recollections can allow feelings to be expressed which have been suppressed, sometimes for years. "Expressions of vulnerability or anger or sadness can become triggers for the memory of the trauma itself, and are therefore forbidden" (Carey, 2006, p. 60).

The title of Session 3 was Finding treasure. The group experienced more warm-ups after the train improvisation: a feelings game called Group Mood (Emunah, 1994, p. 157) which allows participants access to their feelings and emotions. This is helpful to experience the numbness the neuroscientists write about, when the polyvagal nerve which connects the brain to the heart and other organs of the body wakes us up to feeling and connection with self and others. The body-sculpting warm-up is similar, reaching into the somatic work recommended by the trauma theorists and giving opportunities for feelings and moods to be embodied. Individuals work in dyads and take turns to form the other into a statue moving their head, arms, and legs, and suggesting facial expressions representing various feelings. The participant aims to help their partner to be in touch with their bodily self, rather than trying to puzzle things out in their head during the experience (Emunah, 1994, p. 148). The mirror neurons are able to show a participant observer what a body sculpt of anger or surprise looks like, bringing them closer to feeling it themselves. The neuroscience behind these warm-ups gives participants the chance to feel embodied. Because of the shrinking of the hippocampus mentioned earlier in ageing, dementia and PTSD, messages in the brain of fear and anxiety are not always able to reach the decision-making frontal lobe, and so the poor body takes the load of the cold sweats, the heart-racing and dissociated emptiness that results from PTSD.

This warming up phase was a prelude to the finding of treasure, and projection presented a way of bringing joy in the playful "lucky dip" engagement of blindly choosing an object and removing it from a bag. Tanya at first took out a matchbox with which she was unsatisfied, so she had a second opportunity. When she had felt inside and then saw the baboushka doll, she drew it close to her. However, a moment later, she complained that her brain had left her (a complaint she often made, whereupon everyone in the group would help to hunt for it!). Tanya wailed: "It's somewhere in Vienna with the Nazis walking in". Quick as a flash came Ben's rejoinder: "What about - that's not it there, in your hands?" Ben had chosen a great way of helping her to rely on her brain at the same time as noticing the object she had withdrawn. (This was an achievement for Ben, whose dementia was trending towards severe.) Tanya then reflectively explored the smaller versions of the baboushka enclosed inside it, engaging with her memory of a similar doll her father had brought her from Russia, all those years ago.

For Tanya, there were many layers. The baboushka symbolised the layers of embodiment we all share as young children, and it gave her the chance to connect with them in the object, instead of doing so in her frail elderly body which did not allow much movement. Then she told us that her father had brought her a similar doll back from Turkestan where he had been in prison. This was the father she loved, who had rescued his family by arranging their flight to Holland by train, and later to Australia by air. There was additionally the sense that Tanya, a highly intelligent woman, recognised despite her dementia that humans are many-sheathed creatures. Tanya was interested in Jungian psychology and had already reminded us of the subconscious in an earlier session when discussing our group agreement.

David (74) had attended a Catholic boarding school as a child which had a terrible history of child abuse at the time he was in high school (Coote, 2017). He was able, in Session 11 to improvise scenarios from his school life which showed us plainly that he was often hiding from the teaching brothers. He disclosed being physically abused and I questioned in my own mind whether he was sexually abused. He was often evasive, using satire and inappropriate humour to hide feelings. Dramatherapist Craig Haen says of such children: "Boys who have been sexually abused present strong clinical challenges; guarded, evasive, tentative, angry and terribly afraid to trust" (Haen, 2007, p. 250). These characteristics can apply to boys who have been physically abused as well. It is likely that for an elderly adult who has not experienced therapy before, symbolic enactment could have shielded and defended against the distress of memories of the beatings or worse (Jaaniste, 2013).

This is also important in all the arts therapies, so that the person with dementia can feel held in empathic regard, whether there is recall of the trauma or not. If scenes from the life story are played out in dramatherapy, specific attention is needed by the therapist to make sure the person is not re-traumatised, but instead is brought back to the here-and-now with a more balanced sense of the events that occurred long ago. This was the case for David, when he had mimed the role of the boy who was caned at school and hiding from his tormentor. Thorough de-roling from being a young student and naming himself as a 74-year-old man helped him back to the present. A period of reflection, with others recalling unfairness from their school days, brought about a change in mood, and the realisation he had actually been heroic since he had summoned up the courage to complain to the headmaster about physical abuse. The principal then fortunately took him seriously and removed the teacher from that class.

DAVID: I got the cane all the time. So one time I just said "Gee – haven't I had enough?" and he dropped the bloody cane and gave me a belt around the bloody head and one of my mates got up and said "Leave him alone". I turned around and raced out of the classroom and went up to the headmaster and the headmaster came down the next day and said, "This class is dropping Latin and French and taking up geography and history from here on".

STUDENT: Wow.

DAVID: So I copped a belting but anyway I got rid of him. That's a true story too.

JOANNA: So how many strokes of the cane had you had before you said "haven't I had enough?"

DAVID: Oh about three, you know. So, ah, anyway, that's what happened.

JOANNA: It was such a cruel practice, wasn't it?

DAVID: Oh yes, in those days.

BEN: Oh yes.

DAVID: I used to keep a record of the number of strokes of the cane I'd get a week.

BEN: It was a rough gig, that one sometimes.

It is not always possible to help heal past issues of abuse, but there are examples of emotional trauma in this chapter which illustrate a successful return to the present moment, and others in the book which may present the reader with further questions. Often, specific cultural, racial and class considerations can be at the root of trauma, and some of these questions will be addressed in the next chapter. Most individuals discussed are of Anglo-Celtic descent unless their ethnicity is mentioned, such as Tanya's Austrian origins.

Leanne's childhood emotional abuse and Role, Projection and Embodiment

In Chapter 5, the term RPE is explained as a way of reversing Sue Jennings' paradigm of Embodiment, Projection and Role (EPR) and employing it for people with dementia as RPE.

The story of Leanne's childhood trauma at the age of nine and the work we did in several sessions relating to its memory are firmly connected with Sue Jennings' developmental paradigm of EPR (Jennings, 1999).

I learned from staff at the day centre and from her carer that Leanne (70) was angry and had an obsessional memory about ongoing emotional abuse in childhood. In the day centre where the sessions took place, there were other activities Leanne attended where she would share her experience as a nine-year-old. The principal of her primary school had made her stand next to her for weeks at playtime and denied her any play. Leanne to this day had no idea why. In the very first session, where black and white photos were laid out for people to choose and reflect upon, Leanne chose a picture of a young boy walking along in boots that she said were much too big for him. She told us the boy was walking and looking at the ground and was "not a happy chappie". She said, "I think he's feeling a bit subdued at the moment". Leanne knew we would be playing a great deal, and she had been denied playtime for an extended period in primary school. Her mood was very flat. It's hard to play in grown-up boots. Carey (2006) connects the polarities of genuine sadness with overwhelm from earlier trauma: "a split between a state of shut-down where expression of sadness or loss might trigger their own associations of childhood trauma, and the expression of overwhelming feelings when the memory of the trauma surfaced" (p. 34). In that session, Leanne expressed the hope that the group would be "dramatic". At that stage, we had no idea how dramatic the dramatherapy experience would be for her, as we worked throughout with this traumatic memory.

Session 6 was the first time Leanne spoke to us as a group about her experience. These were the words she used to tell us about her story:

> My most live memory (of rage) was when I was about – at school, and one of the teachers, um, decided that she, that I had to stand beside her every lunch time. I could have eaten her – I was so angry for a long time because everybody else went out to play and I had to stand beside that loathsome woman and learn to hate. I'd never learned to hate before.

At this point, we were all in a circle inside a Developmental Transformations (DvT) Magic Box (see Chapter 3, pp. 34–35). We made a circle, and I described a large imaginary soup tureen in the centre, known in DvT terms as an Emotional Soup. I asked the group if there was anything they didn't like or want that they would like to throw into the pot, starting with Leanne. She threw in "a lot of memories … from that woman". Everyone else in the group contributed to the pot, and then I asked what they would like to do with it. Leanne said: "Chuck it out of the window". We eventually carried it out through the door, this imaginary pot, dramatically staggering under its weight, and left it in the garden.

In Session 11, Dealing with Difficult People, I had tried to reverse roles with Leanne. She was all ready to talk about the principal of her school again, and so I asked her to play herself while I played the headmistress. This did not work at all well, and during the interchange, I realised that Leanne, since her dementia was not mild but moderate, could not hold that conversation in role as she did not recognise the difference between "me and not me". I had to close down the discussion and go onto the next person presenting a difficult situation. The Emotional Soup had worked well for Leanne, because we were working with projection; role-play had not been the correct way to deal with the issue. Her last words in the role-play interchange were that she felt very alone. I asked if there was anyone else who had been made to feel alone, and invited them to come and stand next to Leanne. Two of them did so, and I asked her to look at their faces, and tell me about them. She said, "They're all smiling". They were, but it was still difficult for Leanne to calm down after that scene, and I resolved that I would look for an opportunity in a future session to use projection to help with her issue.

Leanne's work in overcoming her traumatic memory

It was not until Session 15 that the moment seemed right to work with Leanne's traumatic memory. The session was called Grief and loss 2. I inevitably give the people I work with the chance before sessions are terminated to deal with their losses. It helps them to mark the ending and leaves the last session of all to be a celebration (see Chapter 8, p. 108).

After a warm-up walking around the room and owning the space, participants took part in an intense trust exercise where they worked in dyads, walking around in turn and leading their partner whose eyes were closed, managing their safety by warning of any obstacles in their path. Once again, this exercise gave people a body awareness through aiming to trust their bodies as well as their guides. Participants connected with themselves somatically before moving into a personal story. Leanne told us why she was angry:

> When I went to school I had a principal in the school who never let me play. Not once. I had to stand beside her and hate her. Can you understand that? Every day. I'd come out. Other people would be playing. All the people in the school were playing except me. I never got to play. She had – she walked beside me all the time and you have no idea how much I hate her. That was all of my freedom. There was just no, no backing out, no way of escaping. It's not fair.

I asked Leanne to show us the drawing she had made (Figure 7.1).

Leanne at eight or nine had been old enough to realise she "didn't have any childhood". This statement showed all of her distress and sense of innocence that had been taken away. I asked the group to help set up a scene where all the chairs were moved out of the way except for one, which was named "Mrs L", and Leanne dressed it up in her least favourite colours. The chair was festooned with black and grey cloths, and Leanne

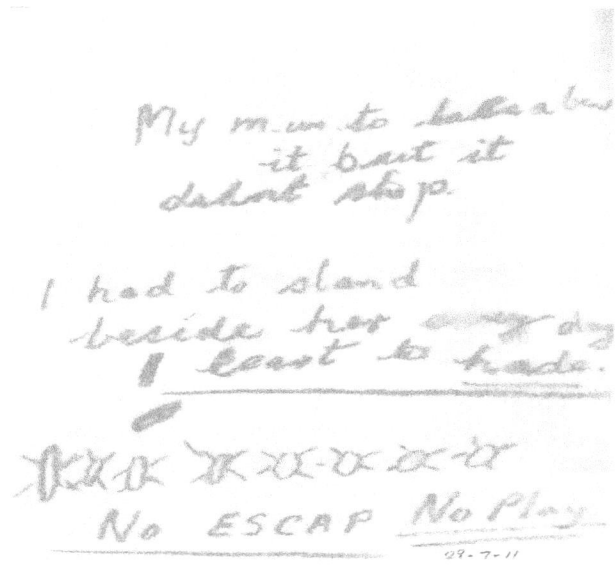

Figure 7.1 Leanne's written and illustrated memory of being emotionally abused at age nine

dressed herself in her favourite colours – green and yellow. She stood right next to the "Mrs L chair" and I asked the group to pull her away so that we could all play together. This was the projection and collaborative activity that might give her the support to deal with this issue.

Others in the group suggested chasings, and chased one other around Mrs L, changing to a game of Stuck in the Mud. Leanne tagged people who then "froze", and frozen participants stood astride, allowing another to crawl through their legs to free them. During the game, participants were shouting at Mrs L – "boo, boo" and "this is fun!"

LEANNE: You're horrid. You're a thorough bastard. I hate you too.
STAFF: I hate you. Hate you. Hate you.
NEIL: You're the worst teacher in the world.
LEANNE: She was, I reckon. It was just appalling. My mum went down and mum was in tears. Just, you know … I was nine.
BEN: Nine was a kid.
STUDENT: That's horrible.
BEN: Horrible.
JOANNA: Have you got anything else you want to say to her?
LEANNE: Mrs L, get out of my hair. I don't want to hear you, see you, smell you, or anything ever again.
JOANNA: Anything else?
LEANNE: I'm glad this is all over.

After about 10 minutes, she decided Mrs. L should go outside, where the Emotional Soup had been discharged some weeks back. One participant said, "She's struggling, she doesn't want to go!" Neil said, "Keep your colours" when it looked as though Leanne was about to leave her green and yellow cloths outside. Others assisting said, "Leanne's the queen of the castle" and "Lock her out the door!". Leanne was relieved to dismiss the teacher; she said she didn't always want to be looking down and feeling miserable. (No one had referred since to her chosen picture in Session 1.) When asked how it felt to take part in the activity, Leanne said, "It was very therapatic (sic)".

Basically, Leanne had been traumatised by childhood cruelty and humiliation in relation to her teacher at school. The forcing of power and control had been still very alive for her in the present with strong affect. Her story was chosen because of this and because it would resonate in the group, as every child has had a humiliating experience, often at school, so others had the potential to identify with her and support her. The participants' willingness to take a role in another person's story indicates those with dementia can still have the capacity to enter the experience of another person in an imaginative and sensitive way (see Chapter 5 on Feeling Intelligence). It may be important to provide more opportunities for people with dementia to do this.

I spoke to her husband/carer husband several times during the following year, and even one year later, Leanne had never once mentioned the traumatic incident again. Leanne may have smoothed over that period of her life like Nicci Gerrard's (2019) mother or it may have sprung back when asked to play as a 70-year-old, who knows. The true story speaks of being blamed for something she didn't understand, singled out and deprived of her playmates, humiliated on behalf of her mother as well as herself. The play Leanne had experienced, the loosening of her limbs and spontaneous fun, had helped her somatically to overcome the trauma response of rigidity and resistance she had before, once this memory surfaced. The "flying cockroach" she had enrolled in during an earlier session had appeared again in her painting – perhaps they were her fellow playmates in the enactment. The songs we sang at the end were "We'll meet again" (Robin & Rainger, 1938) and "Near friends, dear friends" (Watts, 2006), emphasising her experience of being met so warmly by others in the dramatherapy space.

In the following chapter, other stories of grief and loss will be considered, not always born out of trauma. Perhaps we are beginning to understand grief better than was the case for the generation of participants in the present study. It was Leanne who, in Grief and Loss (1) had said how insensitive others could be when they told the bereaved to "get over it". The person with dementia has not only their own loss of memory but also loss of face recognition, words, interests, visitors and much more to cope with compared to those without the diagnosis. Yet the family is there, watching the gradual loss of the person they have known and loved. For dramatherapists, every opportunity counts where we can intervene and help to grieve losses large or small, so that the strain of each addition does not become a weight too unbearable for their clients to carry.

References

Allen, G., Barnard, H., McColl, R., Hester, A. L., Fields, J. A., Weiner, M. F., Ringe, W. K., Lipton, A. M., Brooker, M., McDonald, E., Rubin, C. D., & Cullum, C. M. (2007). Reduced hippocampal functional connectivity in Alzheimer's disease. *Archives of Neurology*, *64*(10), 1482–1487.

American Psychiatric Association. (2013). *Diagnostic and statistical manual of mental disorders* (5th ed.). Author.

Barnes, D. E., Byers, A. L., Gardner, R. C., Seal, K. H., Boscardin, J., & Yaffe, K. (2018). Association of mild traumatic brain injury with or without loss of consciousness with American Veterans. *Journal of the American Medical Association Neurology*, *75*(9), 1055–1061.

Black Dog Institute. (2021). *Post-traumatic stress disorder*. https://www.blackdoginsti tute.org.au/resources-support/post-traumatic-stress-disorder/

Blue Knot Foundation. National Centre of Excellence for Complex Trauma. (2019, December 4). *What is complex trauma?* https://www.blueknot.org.au/Resources/Information/Understanding-abuse-and-trauma/What-is-complex-trauma

Butterworth, B. R. (2018). What World War One taught us about PTSD. *The Conversation*. theconversation.com/what-world-war-i-taught-us-about-ptsd-105613

Carey, L. (Ed.). (2006). *Expressive & creative arts methods for trauma survivors*. Jessica Kingsley Publications.

Clément, J.-P. (2012). Traumatism during childhood and risk of late-onset dementia. *Neuropsychiatrie de l'enfance et de l'adolescence*, *60*, 350–355.

Cook, J. M., & Simiola, V. (2018). Trauma and aging. *Current Psychiatry Reports*, *20*(93), 1–9. https://doi.org/10.1007/s11920-018-0943-6.

Coote, G. (2017, January 20). *Australia's oldest catholic boys' boarding school to formally apologise to sex abuse victims* [Radio broadcast]. ABC. https://abc.net.au/news/2017-01-20/bathurst-school-to-formally-apologise-over-sexual-abuse/8197290

Craftman, A. G., Swall, A., Bakman, K., Grundberg, A., & Hagelin, C. L. (2020). Caring for older people with dementia living past trauma. *Nursing Ethics*, *27*(2), 621–633.

Dementia Australia. (2021). *Causes of dementia*. https://www.dementia.org.au/about-dementia/dementia-research/causes-of-dementia

Emunah, R. (1994). *Acting for real*. Brunner Mazel, Inc.

Flannery, R. B. (2002). Addressing psychological trauma in dementia sufferers. *American Journal of Alzheimer's Disease and Other Dementias*, *17*(5), 281–285.

Gensowski, M., Nielsen, T. H., Nielsen, N. M., Rossin-Slater, M., & Wüst, M. (2019). Childhood health shocks, comparative advantage, and long-term outcomes: Evidence from the last Danish polio epidemic. *Journal of Health Economics*, *66*, 27–36.

Gerrard, N. (2019). *What dementia teaches us about love*. Penguin Random House.

Hachinski, V. (2008). Shifts in thinking about dementia. *Journal of the American Medical Association, 12*, 2172–2173.

Haen, C. (2007). Fear to tread: Play and dramatherapy in the treatment of boys who have been sexually abused. In S. Brooke (Ed.), *The use of creative therapies with sexual abuse survivors* (pp. 235–249). Charles C. Thomas.

Herman, J. L. (1992). *Trauma and recovery*. Basic Books.

International Statistical Classification of Diseases and Related Health Problems (11th ed.: ICD-11. World Health Organisation, 2019).

Jaaniste, E. J. (2013). *Pulled through a hedge backwards: Improving the quality of life of people with dementia through dramatherapy* [Unpublished PhD Thesis]. University of Western Sydney.

Jaaniste, J., & Perry, S. (2021). Art and dramatherapists together consider a multi-modal approach for supporting clients with complex trauma. *JoCAT, 16*(1), 44–54.

Jennings, S. (1999). *Introduction to developmental playtherapy*. Jessica Kingsley Publishers.

Jones, P. (2007). *Drama as therapy: Theory, practice and research* (2nd ed.). Routledge.

Kessler et al. (2018, September 17). Trauma and PTSD in the WHO World Mental Health surveys. *European Journal of Psychotraumatology, 8*(5), 1–18. https://doi.org/10.1080/20008198.2017.1353383

Kivipelto, M., & Solomon, A. (2009). Preventive neurology. On the way from knowledge to action. *Neurology, 73*(3), 168–169.

Lamb, C. (2020). *Our bodies, their battlefield: What war does to women*. William Collins.

Levine, P. (1997). *Waking the tiger: Healing trauma*. North Atlantic Books.

Meziab, O., Kirby, K. A., Williams, B., Yaffe, K., Byers, A. L., & Barnes, D. E. (2014). Prisoner of war status, post-traumatic stress disorder and dementia in older veterans. *Alzheimer's and Dementia, 10*(3), D236–D241.

Porges, S. W. (1997). Emotion: An evolutionary bi-product of the neural regulation of the autonomic nervous system. In C. S. Carter, I. I. Lederhendler, & B. Kirkpatrick (Eds.), *The integrative neurobiology of affiliation* (pp. 62–77). New York Academy of Sciences.

Porges, S. W. (2004). Neuroception: A subconscious system for detecting threats and safety. *Zero to Three, 24*(5), 19–24.

Radford, K., Mack, H. A., Draper, B., Chalkley, S., Daylight, G., Cumming, R., Bennett, H., Delbaere, K, & Broe, G. A. (2015). Prevalence of dementia in urban and regional Australians. *Alzheimer's & Dementia, 11(3)*, 271–279.

Radford,K., Delbaere, K., Draper, B., Mack, H. A., Daylight, G., Cumming, R., Chalkley, S., Minogue, C., & Broe, G. A. (2017). Childhood stress and adversity is associated with late-life dementia in Aboriginal Australians. *American Journal of Geriatric Psychiatry, 25*(10), 1097–1106.

Read Johnson, D. (1987). The role of the creative arts therapies in the diagnosis and treatment of psychological trauma. *The Arts in Psychotherapy, 14*(1), 7–13.

Rehman, Y., Zhang, C., Fernandes, H., Marek, L., Cretu, M., & Parkinson, A. (2020). The extent of the neurocognitive impairment in elderly survivors of war suffering from PTSD: Meta-analysis and literature review. *AIMS Neuroscience, 8*(1), 47–73.

Robin, L., & Rainger, R. (1938). Thanks for the memory [song lyrics]. *Lyrics Depot.* http://www.lyricsdepot.com/shep-fields/thanks-for-the-memory.html

Sethi, D., & Butchart, A. (2017). Violence/intentional injuries, prevention & control. In S. R. Quah (Ed.), *International encyclopaedia of public health* (2nd ed., pp. 351–359). Elsevier Academic Press.

Smith, K., Flicker, L., Lautenschlager, N. T., Almeida, O. P., Atkinson, D., Dwyer, A., & LoGiudice, D. (2008). High prevalence of dementia and cognitive impairment in Indigenous Australians. *Neurology*, *71*(19), 1470–1473.

Snowden, D. (2001). *Aging with grace: What the Nun Study teaches us about leading longer, healthier and more meaningful lives*. Bantam Books.

Stern, L., & Hulko, W. (2016). Historical trauma, PTSD & dementia: Implications for trauma-informed social work. *The Gerontologist*, *56* (Issue Supplement 3), 311.

Tani, Y., Fujiwara, T., & Kondo, K. (2020). Association between adverse childhood experiences and dementia in older Japanese adults. *Journal of the American Medical Association*, *3*(2), e1920740. https://doi.org/10.1001/jamanetworkopen.2019.20740

van der Kolk, B. A. (2002). Posttraumatic therapy in the age of neuroscience. *Psychoanalytic Dialogues*, *12*(3), 381–392. https://doi.org/10.1080/10481881209348674

van der Kolk, B. A. (2014). *The body keeps the score*. Penguin Group.

Vasterling, J. J., Duke, L. M., Brailey, K., Constans, J. I., Allain, A. N., Jr., & Sutker, P. B. (2002). Attention, learning, and memory performances and intellectual resources in Vietnam veterans: PTSD and no disorder comparisons. *Neuropsychology*, *16*, 5–14.

Watts, J. (2006). *A few songs occasioned by the Spirit*. http://jonwattsmusic.com/album/a-few-songs-occasioned

Webb, N. B. (Ed.). (2004). *Mass trauma and violence: Helping families and children cope*. Guilford Press.

Yaffe, K., Vittinghoff, E., Lindquist, K., Barnes, D., Covinsky, K. E., Neylan, T., Kluse, M., & Marmar, C. (2010). Posttraumatic stress disorder and risk of dementia among US veterans. *Archives of General Psychiatry*, *67*(6), 608–613.

Yehuda, R., & LeDoux, J. (2007). Response variation following trauma: A translational neuroscience approach to understanding PTSD. *Neuron*, *56*(1), 19–32.

Chapter 8

Grief and loss in old age

This chapter moves from the area of PTSD and trauma, the results of which many people still face in old age, to grief and loss, sometimes heavily connected to earlier trauma, and how the mourning can take place through ritualised interventions of dramatherapy. For many people with dementia, they have faced the shock of the diagnosis initially, and then the often-scattered memories from early life which are reminders of traumatic experiences. They have also lost loved ones, and if in a facility for the aged, may have few or no visitors at all.

In a novel about an elderly man who is feeling the oncoming scourge of dementia, Sara Gruen writes of the grief of memory loss in a nursing home. This man led an adventurous, risk-taking younger life as a vet in a travelling circus and later a more settled one in the suburbs, working in an animal clinic. He describes how he feels himself sliding into an ill-defined mind space. He says that his brain feels like the cosmos where the air is getting ever thinner, but does not disappear into nothing. He has the sense that something "out there" is awaiting him and then finds himself sliding in its direction once more with his mouth wide open (Gruen, 2006).

Gruen brings an honesty to the character which may be modelled on someone she knew well. There are so many losses in dementia: not only the loss of memory, but also sensory loss, weight loss, the deprivation of independence, semantic loss in language and many more. Some of the losses are considered here.

Sensory loss

Hearing impairment

Hearing impairment in older people often precedes dementia. A case-control study was published 30 years ago on this new topic of a possible connection between deficient hearing and the onset of dementia (Uhlmann et al., 1989). Little further research had been carried out on this phenomenon up until eight years ago (Lin & Albert, 2014). More recently though, hearing

DOI: 10.4324/9781003186328-8

loss has been found to contribute to not only social isolation, which is a more obvious result of hearing impairment, but also in some cases, a deficit of serotonin (Keesom & Hurley, 2020). This is a neuro-moderator which can affect pathways to the brain as well as the auditory system. Serotonin is involved in mood and affect generally, and the lack of it can not only play a role in depression and anxiety but also have an effect in the understanding of speech, especially in situations where there is other sound going on (Keesom & Hurley, 2020). In such cases, the loss experienced by the person with dementia could feel like double jeopardy.

Sense of smell

One of the senses not widely recognised as dementia-affected is the sense of smell. While undertaking my fieldwork, I had not come across details of this deficit in my reading and imagined that a smelling game would be ideal for my group in Session 13. The main theme of this session, entitled The joys and woes of memory, was a guessing game to identify various scents, and I was hoping their aromas would bring back memories. Ten small, numbered muslin bags filled with herbs and powders were suspended on strings and participants were given notebooks and pencils to identify the scents against each number. Very few words were inscribed in the notebooks or in the reflection period after the game, and it became obvious that I had set up these intrepid and loyal individuals to fail in their task. After the session, of course, having discovered how few scents could be named, my belated research on olfactory deficits and their role in predicting the later onset of dementia (Wilson et al., 2009) revealed this aspect of the condition. Fortunately, however, something significant was salvaged for at least one participant – an important memory for Neil of fruit in his mother's kitchen when he was a little boy carried over until the next session. The memory prompted a roleplay in the 14th session on grief and loss (Jaaniste, 2013). This memory is expanded upon in a vignette later in the chapter.

Weight loss

There are several reasons for loss of weight in people with dementia. People may lose the ability to recognise the meals they are offered. Some people become unable to swallow properly. They may forget to or refuse to eat or have difficulty swallowing. For others, medication that may not necessarily be prescribed for dementia, but is given for other co-morbid conditions, may have side effects which impact on appetite. They may have disrupted leptin levels caused by the disease, so that they are not being informed by natural hormonal weight control signals that they have not had enough to eat (Franx et al., 2017). From a taste enjoyment point of view as well as nutritionally, there is considerable loss as they age and in particular when they have dementia. Even unhealthy weight gain may be a loss of sorts, where they over-eat, and cannot recognise their body shape anymore.

Physical pain

Pain is described as an "unpleasant sensory and emotional experience associated with actual or potential tissue damage or described in terms of such damage" (Merskey & Bogduk, 1994, as cited in Schofield, 2018, i7). It is assessed as acute when it is caused by trauma or an injury, or chronic when it has a duration of not less than three months. So many people who are experiencing dementia are also feeling the physical pain of rheumatism or arthritis, bruising as a result of falls and inexplicable headaches and digestive problems. They are feeling the loss of their flexible and healthy body of earlier years as sclerotic problems develop and the physical body dries out and becomes more rigid. As well as this, we (as I need to include myself here) find ourselves catching a glimpse of ourselves in the mirror and failing to recognise the person who looks back. Is that wrinkled person with the grey hair and the thickened waist really me? I tell people I like my wrinkles, but on some days, this is far from the case! Although I would never have plastic surgery or Botox, it is discouraging to find some new loose skin hanging around the neck. We carry ourselves at all our ages into the final years, so bear aspects of our souls that are forever young, with the outside appearance belying the internal child or 20-year-old.

Loss of language

Communication in language is affected in people ageing normally as well as in people with dementia, but for most people with dementia, language loss is a problem, especially as the disease progresses. Problems with word retrieval can result in forgetting names of friends and relatives, leading to confusing family relationships, and can exacerbate lack of recognition of loved ones (Miller, 2002). Difficulties with expression can leave the person imprisoned in their feelings and thoughts, relying on others to try to understand what they mean (Edberg, 2000). It is important to encourage immigrant participants to speak in their first language when the English words get stuck, as the original language will be more accessible to them.

Loss of independence

If we are elderly and do not have dementia, we may be on a conscious journey which helps us to resolve the changes in our life. Jungian thinker Helen Luke believes that when we reach a certain stage in our lives, we begin to realise that our "much prized reasoning" (Luke, 2010, p. 98) does not necessarily lead to happiness. We do become aware that we join a oneness with all that is in the world, including its suffering. However, for someone whose situation brings existential anxieties when cognitive faculties are failing them, the path is not as smooth and any burden of suffering is more difficult to bear.

Working in mental health over the last many years, I have been inspired by John Bowlby's (1980) work on grief and loss in mental health. Bowlby writes about the "prolonged absence of conscious grieving" (p. 138) which can take place in mental illness. Bowlby mentions that during psychotherapy, ill-defined symptoms which occur, occasionally after breakdown, are found to derive from normal mourning, although they are oddly disconnected from the original loss which led to them. His work is significant in connection with people with dementia. He considers that a delayed reaction to the grief which the person experiences at the time of loss can impact on future losses. Thus, if the first loss is not dealt with in some way, through ritual or interpersonal connection, the second one is exacerbated. There can be a masked grief reaction where people can experience symptoms and habits which they do not understand or which cause problems, but the fact that these are related to the first grief remains hidden. This is why it is important for us to consider the grieving of people with dementia, whose losses before and after their diagnosis follow quickly one after the other. This situation has ramifications for training staff and families, as such recognition shows the importance of connecting with them over their multiple reasons for grieving.

As individuals age, they naturally experience loss. The resulting grief can affect their feeling life, such as isolation or depression, their physicality because of lack of mobility and pain, or changes in environment such as living alone or being moved into care. Alongside these losses, they are losing their memories, words and sense of self. There are many models of grieving which can help people, but some of the cognitive difficulties that come with dementia can confuse the process. A review of the literature indicates that health workers and family members of people with dementia find it difficult to talk about grieving with them or under-estimate their capacity for doing so (Doka, 2004; Rentz et al., 2004–5). All of our models of grief and mourning presuppose integrated cognitive ability and Rentz et al. ask, should we broaden the models to include self-loss, and try to look at grieving through a new lens? Doka (2004) believes grief is a "constant companion to Alzheimer's disease and related dementias" (p. 20). He explains various ways in which families and carers can connect with the disenfranchised grief of the person with dementia, such as putting together albums of photographs and showing videos. I submit that the arts therapies are routinely able to do this in a very personal and sometimes intimate way, seeking their expression and engaging with the person's creativity, as well as using other methods such as roleplay and improvisation.

Dramatherapy and grief

Dramatherapist Alida Gersie (1991) tells us how storytelling and creative arts activities can remind people of narratives of mourning and their hidden grief, and her words are particularly relevant here. For the elderly people she describes below, whose care workers or family are sometimes so busy with the practical solutions for fading memory, depression and loss of skills of their person with dementia, conversations surrounding the real and some-times heartbreaking issues of grief and loss do not happen.

> Numerous reasons may have led us to keep our grief under tight control and therefore to wait incessantly, or we may have been forced to run away from our mourning and thereby never rest again. When we are thus knotted up inside ourselves, preoccupied with words spoken and deeds done or words unspoken and deeds undone, we may at last seek help, or help may be offered.
>
> (Gersie, 1991, p. 232)

This "grief (kept) under tight control" can be an unwelcome stress and even a kind of inner paralysis for people who have received a dementia diagnosis. Elsewhere I have written about the importance of closure in a dramatherapy group, which has particular significance for people with dementia. The reference is also relevant for Bowlby's model of grief reaction delay:

> From the first day onward there should be some kind of ritual ending for the session. This could be a song, a verse, a gesture – the group may find a way of providing this if the therapist does not. These people are living the last years of their lives, and endings are important; mark-ing them will help with their grief process, as noted with the 'funeral table' example (Chin, 1996). A period of reflection, as shown in previous examples, can connect imaginary scenes with participants' lives and is existentially important.
>
> (Jaaniste, 2011, p. 66)

Chin's funeral table will appear again in one of the vignettes below.

The bereavement exclusion

The diagnostic manual, DSM 4 (American Psychiatric Association (APA), 1952) included a bereavement exclusion (BE) with regard to the diagnosis of major depression. It stated that if someone had depression as a result of the death of a loved one for up to two months after the death, it did not need to be diagnosed as such, even if severe. There was a highly contro-versial change which appeared between the DSM 4 (APA, 1952) and the

DSM 5 (APA, 2013). It was generally believed among critics that removal of the BE would turn natural human grief into a medical diagnosis and the over-prescription of anti-depressant medication would follow (Pies, 2014). Theorists who support the DSM-5's view say there is no reasonable basis for leaving aside people from a diagnosis of depression merely because it becomes apparent when someone close to them has died. Though bereavement-related grief and major depression share some features, they are distinct and distinguishable conditions. The recognition of deep depression in the context of recent bereavement needs clinical experience and wise judgment. However, if severe depression is diagnosed, the person with dementia has every right to appropriate medication and care.

Those thinkers arguing in favour of the BE (Iglewicz et al., 2013; Pies, 2014; Zachar et al., 2017) have noted that the BE will be and has proved to be a helpful decision. Zachar and his colleagues in particular consider that the terrible predictions that getting rid of it would result in a flood of cases of depression and unnecessary prescriptions have not proven correct. In their view, this 2013 change better clarifies the difference between normal grief and a major depressive disorder and was a significant improvement. I include this in the chapter, not because arts and other therapists need to have our eyes constantly on the diagnosis of participants and the manuals where they are listed – we don't. We need to apply our skills to the whole person and the inner spark that makes them human. I include it because these people can often suffer from depression, and to emphasise the importance of our awareness of this circumstance. Vignettes from three separate sessions follow where grief occurred and was addressed. The first two are from my community fieldwork: firstly, the seventh in a group of eight sessions, followed by a two-week break and secondly, the 14th of 16 sessions. I often work with grief and loss when a program is about to end. The third is a session with a different group in a residential care home.

Session 7 – Grief and loss

The session began with a loss straight away – Leanne had arrived with a patch covering one eye, as she had a torn retina and could not see from her left eye. She said she felt "written off". It struck me that we are often seen through the eyes of others, especially family members, and how aptly this expression suited the consequences of the dementia diagnosis.

I told them about the session and that the day's theme was grief and loss.

JOANNA: It's not about someone slapping you on the back and telling you to get over it. That is not a recipe for dealing with grief and loss, is it? Would you agree?

NEIL: Yeah.

LEANNE: Actually, it's damn ridiculous to say 'get over it' because it doesn't help.
JOANNA: It doesn't help.
DAVID: Not at all.

The first warm-up was a trust exercise in pairs, where each person was led around the room by their partner, and either had a blindfold or kept their eyes closed. The risk level, physically or psychologically, was not as high as it would have been earlier in the program, as the group had built a degree of trust in one another. The session chronologically followed Session 6, The joys and woes of memory, when participants had walked through installations representing stages of development in their lives, described in Chapter 3. By engaging in this practice, they had found ideas and experiences in common. The group spent a long time talking about how they felt to walk around being led by another person and what safety meant to them. For most participants, their safety was intact when being steered around, except for David, who was uncomfortable and was glad not to have a blindfold. He may have been unwilling to let go of an experience that belonged to the time before his diagnosis, in order to accept what was ahead. (I could identify as I am familiar with that kind of stubbornness in relinquishing my previous abilities due to physical deterioration, etc.)

I encouraged the group to pass around words about loss as they threw the ball to each other. Some of the words spoken were "aloneness", "emptiness" and "loss of work" (Neil), "loss of my dog" (David), and "loss of comfort" and feeling "threatened, angry and a bit lost" (Leanne). We talked about some of these shared feelings. Leanne was particularly upset, because she already felt off-colour because of her eye. When I mentioned that I would tell them a tale, she pleaded, "Tell me a story, tell me a story". I then narrated Ulu and the Breadfruit Tree (Gersie & King, 1990, p. 237). The Hawaiian story concerns Ulu, a father who sacrifices his life on the instruction of the god Mo'o during a meditation at the temple, when he learns this helps his sick son. Before he dies, he asks his wife to bury his body in the garden. A breadfruit tree grows overnight from his burial place, producing fruit which saves his son's life when his mother encourages him to eat it.

After the narration, there were a few comments and a general reluctance to take on a role in performing the story. Neil was very keen and took on the role of Ulu, and David, the sick son. One of the art therapy students took on the role of the mother, Ulu's wife, and a staff member took the role of the breadfruit tree. I re-told the tale as they performed it.

In the reflection period after the performance, Neil said that after playing the role of the person who had died and was buried, being buried in the earth after he himself died was an option he could live with. Interestingly, he said he would be going back into the earth: "I sort of liked that, the strange way that I would, that my body would be part of this soil again".

I had provided a grief table and some flowers (Chin, 1996), and everyone was invited to place a flower there and say a person's name in their memory. David placed a flower there for his twin brother, who was killed in an aeronautical accident. He said, "He's, ah, been a pilot as well. He was in the Australian acrobatic team touring Russia in a competition. It was special. Could do outside loops and inside loops". Peter remembered all those who had died in war. Noel said, "Let's put it this way, I often had conflict with my father, um, but I have a sense of him being around a bit like the play, that he is around in some form or another". The Japanese art therapy student laid a flower on the table for people far from Australia who had died. Leanne said she had not lost anyone, but she was having problems with her vision, so we placed flowers on the table for her wounded eye, and for regeneration. There was a strong sense that the story of Ulu had encouraged the participants to express their grief and that Leanne, with the loss of sight in one eye, had been able to be comforted somewhat by others' thoughts and actions in the session.

Session 14 – Future wants and needs

This session, although not themed as a grief and loss meeting, directly followed the session where the participants had interacted in the smelling game mentioned earlier in this chapter. The session had a bumpy beginning, as Leanne's husband had gone away without telling her where he was going. This could have been forgotten information. Neil had felt "locked in" during the week and David in contrast was "off the leash" as he had got away from his wife and gone on a skiing trip with his buddies. He kept asking Ben what school he had been to, and Ben's body language changed and his speech became awkward, as his childhood and adolescence had been difficult. Paul was missing, as he had experienced a fall during the week, and I was wondering if he would come back, so my concentration was failing me. After playing a game of Fruit Bowl (Farmer, 2012, p. 3) and warming up a little, Neil said suddenly, in relation to the smelling game the previous week: "it wasn't about the actual little parcels you created but it went to another stage". And then: "it sort of shifted away from that smell to … I wasn't thinking about fruit, ordinary things like that - I was thinking about my mother". It turned out that the smell of the orange in the muslin bag the week before had reminded Neil of a particular occasion when she was cutting up fruit in the kitchen and had playfully chased him around the room when he sneaked pieces from the kitchen bench.

The game we had just played had warmed people up to some extent, but we needed more warm-ups if we were to dramatise Neil's memory. We played two games where participants used flexible strength: one involved pushing their palms against a partner's hands while grounding themselves with legs apart, while the other was a mini tug of war with an imaginary rope. We then played a quick game of Cat and Mouse (Farmer, 2012, p. 12), both games acting as a preparation for Neil's recollection of his mother's playfulness in the kitchen of his memory.

Neil told us he believed himself to be six or seven years old in this kitchen scene and helped us set up the room accordingly. He seated himself at the "kitchen table", where his mum was preparing the fruit (probably apples). Ben thought there should be a stove, Neil agreed, and Ben was given the role of the stove. Was there a window? I asked this question and the addition of the window was accompanied by Neil's direction: "Get up here, David". Then Neil invited Leanne to be his mum and she agreed. I knew from her experience earlier in the program that the role would not be easy for her, as her dementia was not of the mild variety and with moderate dementia, it was unlikely she would know how to engage with a role, especially in someone else's drama. However, Neil gave her directions on all she needed to do at the kitchen table, and she added her own self-direction – that the audience needed to see her face, which showed confidence in taking her position in the play space. There was some gentle admonishment from her as Neil snuck a few invisible pieces of fruit and she called him a naughty boy and chased him around the table. Far from concealing his action, he was merely giggling and singing out "you won't catch me!" once he had the fruit safely in his hand.

Ben's reflection on the scene was that "those things just don't happen in houses". This may or may not have been a comment about his own house, but a little later, he said, "I'd like to encourage people to do these things" (perhaps so that they could visit past memories). David commented on the homely atmosphere and how, as his role as the window, he had liked looking into a happy home. After de-roling, Leanne said "Oh, it's very nice and cosy". Perhaps she had played the playful person she wished she'd had in her profession of teacher, and more generally as an adult.

When Neil was asked what his adult self would say to his childhood self, he said: "you're a very lucky boy to have a mum who was playful". He said he was "a bit teary" in the scene, and also responding to "the loss of Mum".

In the grief and loss session the following week, when asked to choose a twig from among a group of small branches, and incorporate it in a painting, Neil depicted the branch with its blossoms released towards the sky. In a group invitation for all participants to speak words about grief and loss, he said of his mother, "I thought I would have you for ever" and "letting me go". His picture (shown as Figure 8.1) represents the bringing together of the kitchen drama from the week before with the memory of his mother. There is a patch of sunlight on the terracotta tiles underneath the painting, where Neil is still walking the earth where he is comfortable about being buried when he dies.

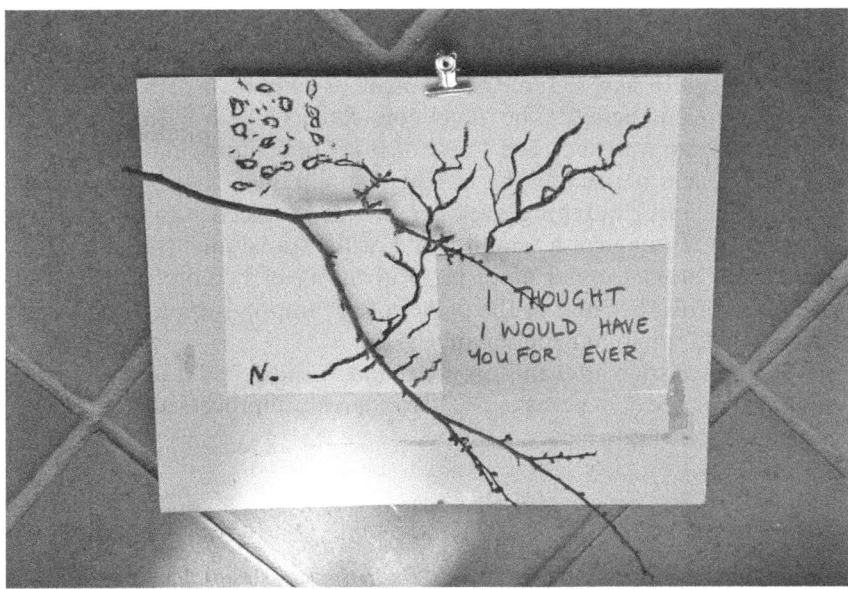

Figure 8.1 Neil's art work in honour of his mother

Session at a local residential care home

Unlike the stories from the vignettes above, the following incident took place in a residential care home in the second session of a program that ran for 10 weeks. Elspeth (89), a woman with mild dementia, arrived in the room with a headache, perhaps as the result of a dream the previous night which she revealed early in the session. Elspeth was in a wheelchair and two others in the group were not ambulant either, so we warmed up with some seated ball-throwing and arm movement activities, and I asked her if she would like to improvise the dream. She narrated that she had died and was observing her life from the sky above. She was experiencing loss, in the sense that she had regrets about her earlier life and blamed herself for some of the ways she had dealt with life's difficulties. One of these was abandonment on board ship on a long journey to Australia with her mother in her teenage years (Jaaniste, 2011). She chose someone to play her adolescent self and others played the ship's captain and her mother. These participants, unlike Elspeth, were able to move around. She told us that her mother spent most of the voyage playing deck quoits with the ship's captain or sitting at his table for meals, while she sat elsewhere. She felt the ship was going to "the land that never was".

Elspeth had probably never told her mother how unfair this felt, and as she watched the improvisation of the deck quoits game, she felt "hope-less". She experienced having failed as a younger person, and this was one of many other occasions where she said she had done so. I asked her to select another person to stand alongside her. She chose the care worker, whom I asked to play the role of an angel, as I knew Elspeth to be someone with angelic beliefs. The angel connected Elspeth with Elspeth the dreamer as she watched. The sense of lost opportunity and death anxiety became less painful as she was held simultaneously by her youthful self and an angel watching over her life. It provided the others in the group with an image of a "smooth end of life transition" (Jaaniste, 2011, pp. 21–22). She accepted more hopeful facets of her life in the reflection afterwards, because of the power of the improvisation and her own strongly held spiritual belief in angels.

Elspeth died soon after this program had finished, and it is possible that this holistic sense of hope, as opposed to a largely unprocessed grief, accompanied her in her passing.

References

American Psychiatric Association. (1952). *Diagnostic and statistical manual of mental disorders* (4th ed.). Author

American Psychiatric Association. (2013). *Diagnostic and statistical manual of mental disorders* (5th ed.). Author.

Bowlby, J. (1980). *Attachment and loss. Vol.3: Loss, sadness & depression*. Hogarth Press.

Chin, C. (1996). Sounding board. Reconstructing the self with drama and creative arts therapies. *American Journal of Alzheimer's Disease, 11*(1), 36–42.

Doka, K. J. (2004). Grief, multiple loss and dementia. *Cruse Bereavement Care, 29*(3), 15–20.

Edberg, A. (2000). Assessment by nurses of mood, general behaviour and functional ability in patients with dementia receiving nursing home care. *Scandinavian Journal of Caring Sciences, 14*, 52–61.

Farmer, D. (2012). *101 more drama games and activities*. CreateSpace.

Gersie, A. (1991). *Storymaking in bereavement: Dragons fight in the meadow*. Jessica Kingsley.

Gersie, A., & King, N. (1990). *Storymaking in education and therapy*. Jessica Kingsley.

Gruen, S. (2006). *Water for elephants*. Allen & Unwin.

Franx, B. A. A., Arnoldussen, I. A. C., Kiliaan, A. J., & Gustafson, D. R. (2017). Weight loss in patients with dementia: Considering the potential impact of pharmacotherapy. *Drugs Aging, 34*(6), 425–436.

Iglewicz, A., Seay, K., Zetumer, S. D., & Zisook, S. (2013). The removal of the bereavement exclusion in the DSM-5: Exploring the evidence. *Current Psychiatry Reports, 15*, article 413.

Jaaniste, J. (2011). Dramatherapy and spirituality in dementia care. *Dramatherapy, 33*(1), 16–27.

Jaaniste, E. J. (2013). *Pulled through a hedge backwards: Improving the quality of life of people with dementia through dramatherapy* [Unpublished PhD Thesis]. University of Western Sydney.

Keesom, S. M., & Hurley, L. M. (2020). Silence, solitude and serotonin: Neural mechanisms linking hearing loss and social isolation. *Brain Sciences*, *10*(6), 367. Retrieved from https://www.ncbi.nlm.nih.gov/pmc/articles/PMC7349698/

Lin, F. R., & Albert, M. (2014). Hearing loss and dementia: Who is listening? *Aging and Mental Health*, *18*(6), 671–673.

Luke, H. (2010). *Old age*. Lindisfarne Books.

Merskey, H., & Bogduk, N. (1994). Classification of chronic pain: Descriptions of chronic pain syndromes and definitions of pain terms. IASP Press.

Miller, L. (2002). Effective communication with older people. *Nursing Standards*, *17*(9), 45–50.

Pies, R. (2014). The bereavement exclusion and DSM-5: An update and commentary. *Innovations in Clinical Neuroscience*, *11*(7–8), 19–22.

Rentz, C., Krikorian, R., & Keys, M. (2004–5). Grief and mourning from the perspective of the person with a dementing illness: Beginning the dialogue. *Omega*, *50*(3), 165–179.

Schofield, P. (2018). The assessment of pain in older people: UK national guidelines. *Age and Ageing*, *47*, i1–i22.

Uhlmann, R. F., Larson, E. B., Koepsell, T. D., & Duckert, L. G. (1989). Relationship of hearing impairment to dementia and cognitive dysfunction in older adults. *Journal of the American Medical Association*, *261*(13), 1916–1919.

Wilson, R. S., Arnold, S., Schneider, J. A., Boyle, P. A., Buchman, A. S., & Bennett, D. A. (2009). Olfactory impairment in presymptomatic Alzheimer's disease. *Annals of the New York Academy of Sciences*, *1170*, 730–735. doi: 10.1111/j.1749-6632.2009.04013.x

Zachar, P., First, M. B., & Kendler, K. S. (2017). The bereavement exclusion debate in the DSM 5: A history. *Clinical Psychological Science*, *5*(5), 890–906.

Chapter 9

The mystery of death

The reader may gain surprising information about how little of a meaningful nature is discussed by elders in nursing homes or palliative care when close to death. Clients' questions may range from this spiritual reassurance to regrets about past failures or omissions, fear of death and concern for those left behind. However, through artistic means, it is possible to inspire participants through other's words and their own to approach the end of life with equanimity. Even with people with dementia poetic text may bring a non-denominational and relevant window onto the mystery of death. Examples of poems for fear of death, grief at death and concern for those left behind are included. Suggestions are made in the chapter about suitable interventions.

Leading on from the previous chapter on grief and loss in old age and particularly for people with dementia, this chapter concerns itself with death and the preparation, sometimes spiritual, for the end of life. It calls on literature and poetry, and the value of speaking, hearing and writing poetry in dramatherapy groups. Whereas the research into grief and loss is well-documented and there is a strong awareness in the aged care field that they are issues needing to be dealt with, there is little research on assisting people with dementia in the face of approaching death and the developmental needs of people in the last life stages.

In the previous chapter, we considered how grief and loss can be addressed through dramatherapy. Relevant interventions were introduced with the potential to engage people with dementia in getting in touch with their losses and finding some light within them, even if only to unburden themselves to some extent from unfinished business. Associated with grief and loss is not only the physical deterioration of the body in a society which lauds youth and their healthy, supple bodies. Connected also is the prospect of their journey towards death, and this journey is a normal topic to consider for any human being as we near the end of life.

Life review and reminiscence therapy are also relevant to consideration of loss. People with mild and moderate dementia are no different from the rest of us in wanting to deal with sadness and regret as we reflect on

DOI: 10.4324/9781003186328-9

our approaching death. It can be a different matter for people with severe dementia and this is indeed the case when they are close to death. This chapter will deal with this last stage first and foremost. People whose symptoms are at this stage are often in palliative care and bedridden when nearing death, but can still benefit from hearing poetry and song once they can no longer read. The chapter will then show how the poetry of others and their own work can help the elderly and those with mild or moderate dementia.

Life review

Life review is a developmental activity which has been recognised by psychotherapists and structured in various ways to help people process thoughts about past lived experiences. It often involves going back to significant events in a life and discussing the meaning of these special moments. When people are younger, there can be more critical analysis involving dates and places, but when working with older people, there is often a need for visual stimulus in the form of imagery and metaphor to engage them in reminiscence therapy. Techniques that can be used include marking the ages of the client using the following as springboards to working together: photographs, diaries, letters, music and food sometimes provided by the family. The person with dementia is encouraged to share and describe important personal events. Similar techniques were employed in the dramatherapy session in Chapter 3, where installations depicting childhood, adolescence, working life, marriage, children and grandchildren are used as markers, in order to evoke memories.

Feil and de Klerk-Rubin (2012) describe their validation method (VM) as an approach that can be helpful to therapists of all persuasions by offering solution-based activities to further communication with people who have memory loss. They encourage acceptance of people with dementia, using techniques of touching and reminiscence. Applying empathic, non-judgmental listening, they aim to improve self-esteem and provide emotional release. Research conducted by Feil (1990; 2012) and Kohn (1993) shows that an additional advantage of the use of VM with elderly people is a finding of decreased caregiver burnout.

Arts therapies and palliative care

In her article on meaning-making in palliative care, dramatherapist Rebecca Redhouse quotes the Help the Hospices Guide for the Arts Therapies website with the following words:

> There now exists a substantial body of evidence for the impact of the arts in healthcare. They provide a more positive experience for patients and users, encourage the upkeep of healthcare premises, improve

clinical outcomes, make training and development more effective, improve communication, support staff and engage local communities in hospice care.

(as cited in Redhouse, 2015)

Creative arts therapists can assist families who are supporting their dying relatives, palliative care teams, and also patients through the bereavement process (Gallagher, 2013). Redhouse points out in her in-depth case study applying dramatherapy to her hospice work that there is very little palliative care research in the literature on dramatherapy. She herself uses spectrograms and dramatic distancing to bring her clients' life story narratives into being, consolidated for them in a biographical book collated by herself as the therapist.[1] There are other resources for those who work in the area, and dramatherapist Alida Gersie has written a very helpful book for therapists who want to bring stories about bereavement to families and their loved ones (Gersie, 1991). Much of the contribution to creative arts therapy in research has been carried out in music therapy (Hartley & Payne, 2008), art therapy and dance-movement therapy (DMT).

Music therapy has been offered to people in palliative care over the past 30 years. For people with dementia, it brings back memories that were laid down early in life, and has been found to enhance communication and spiritual experiences (Salmon, 2001; Warth et al., 2014). In a randomised control study in 2015, receptive music therapy was used to help elderly people in palliative care to express feelings, enhance relaxation and increase well-being. The results of the investigation showed that fatigue was diminished and well-being improved, on the basis of self-assessment (Warth et al., 2015).

Art therapy also has a substantial history of working well with people who have dementia. Dennes and Gilchrist (2005), in their chapter on art therapy with the institutionalised elderly, say that the intervention of art therapy in facilities for the elderly has over the years given recipients a chance to meaningfully bring together a lifetime of experiences. Their work is informed by Byers (1995) and Wilks and Byers (1992), who recommend the use of objects in order to give the person with dementia the sense of human touch, and their view that "empathy, warmth and caring for the client" is of paramount importance (Dennes & Gilchrist, 2005, p. 36). They also value the honouring of individuality and the significance of counter-transference for the therapist, understanding the inevitability of their client's death in the near future, as well as fears for their own and loved ones' deaths. Art therapist Simon Bell (2019) writes about his research in palliative care which demonstrates that art therapy gives people with dementia the opportunity "to explore meaning-making and spirituality". He tells the reader: "In the 16 years I worked for my local hospice I witnessed countless occasions when patients described and reflected on spiritual needs in the context of the art therapy I offered" (p. 18).

Working with researchers and carers when offering art therapy to someone with dementia in relationship with their carer, Honig et al. (2019) were able to see how their art-making represented transitional objects between the client's connection and disassociation. They observed the carer gifting their person with dementia with transient instances of interconnection with themselves. They noticed and listened as a piece of art facilitated the weaving together of threads of relationship between the client and their carer.

Dance-movement therapists Dillenbeck and Hammond-Meiers (2009) have made a study of the role of the DMT practitioner, which can be applied to dramatherapy and other therapies when assisting those at the end of their lives. Their detailed research of dying people's needs at the end of life through the participation of their caregivers illustrates the sensitive role of the therapist. Their research explores the experiences and needs of dying individuals and their caregivers, considering its implications for applied practice in palliative care. They refer to Kübler-Ross' (1969) five stages of grief that people may go through in the process of dying (denial, anger, bargaining, depression and acceptance). They write about our culture, which values motion and production and argue instead for approaching the client from a place of stillness, listening to the body of the person who is dying, since death happens "at a cellular level" (Dillenbeck & Hammond-Meiers, 2009, p. 109). They are aware of the possible isolation of the person who is dying. Along with the other practitioners of arts therapies, the therapist as witness is a role they value. They recommend unconditional positive regard for the person, the possibility of mirroring gestures and the significance of listening when verbal communication is limited. All of these practices are particularly relevant to work with people with severe dementia.

Severe dementia

What is a good death for people with dementia, especially when it comes from a diagnosis of severity of the disease? This question is so difficult to answer, as the person with dementia may have had some idea pre-diagnosis that is no longer possible to express and the family may have their own ideas of what "good" means here. It is important to remember, too, that there may be no family or friend to guide the care home or hospital when the person dies. Possible answers to the question of what constitutes a good death may include the attributes of dying with dignity, being treated respectfully, having one's wishes for the end of life partially met; however, these characteristics may not be available to people with dementia in any of its forms. Small et al. (2007), like the dance-movement therapists quoted above, make the point that our society puts a high value on "doing" rather than "being" in the here-and-now. This leads to the manner of our death being connected with ratings of accomplishment and success. Are we lucky enough (or even clever enough, according to society) to die in our sleep, or musing in an armchair after a solid day's work and a good meal? Are we capable or balanced enough to die peacefully in the face of the pain and misery of a terminal illness? For people with dementia, "a good death" may not be possible.

We know that staff in any retirement village with a nursing home attached can expect people there to die quite frequently; yet the matter of death is rarely spoken about there, even in a palliative care situation where the expectation of a terminal outcome is already known. This is despite the fact that, apart from our birth, our death is one of the most important events that any of us experience. This lack of attention to such conversations is unfortunate, since for many people the discussions or even small references that can occur before it happens can assist by bringing an outcome of a good death.

In some communities, rituals around death may be prescribed in culture and include familiar traditions and customs. Death may occur in the homes of extended families where the person has always lived. If they are in a care home in a first-world country though, there can be misunderstandings for nursing home staff of different traditions. Anne-Mei The (2008) writes about such a case in Holland. On their last visit to their loved one in the home, a South American family from Suriname performed a ritual in order to resolve a problem at the bed of their relative Mrs Sharloo, who had dementia and was close to death. A few days later, it was obvious that she really was dying, so carers phoned the family. The staff looked at her files and realised she was a Christian and that she had seen the pastor and had enjoyed church previously. Undeterred, when the dying Mrs Sharloo called for her children, Surinamese staff from other units came to the bed representing her family. They told her in Surinamese to "go to the other side" and asked her to protect them when she arrived in their traditional home of the dead. The main Surinamese carer laid her out in the traditional manner and waited for the family to come. As far as the caring staff were concerned, Mrs Sharloo had received the proper rituals, whatever was written in the notes about her religion (The, 2008).

In many developed countries, people with dementia choose to stay in their homes for as long as they can, receiving community care. This means that once the families and carers can no longer manage to support them, they enter residential care with more frailty and less cognitive understanding than they did in earlier times. Sometimes protected by well-intentioned staff, the end of life is not discussed. Yet despite their vulnerability, a lack of understanding of the person's potential agency needs to be recognised. It is argued that the practice of withholding information, however well-intentioned, contrasts with findings suggesting that full disclosure is generally beneficial to patients and relatives. Some evidence indicates that not only do residents want to be told about their imminent death, but they would prefer to know in advance when possible so that they can have time to say goodbye. If we try to suppress conversations about death, we forfeit the ability to deal with the questions about the meaning of life that it inevitably brings forward (Mannix, 2017).

A study was carried out by Alftberg et al. (2018) in seven nursing homes in southern Sweden, to explore assistant nurses' experience of conversations about the end of life and dying within the framework of their palliative care in the homes. One of the nurses found the experience too draining to talk about. Another said she could not talk about it until a question came from the patient: "Am I going to die here?" The nurse told the woman that as she was healthy right now, she would be advised not to think about such things. The nurse realised only later that she had shut down an important conversation, and should have started by asking her patient what her own thoughts were about dying (Alftberg et al., 2018).

In my own experience of working as an assistant nurse in a care home in my earlier life, no matter how severe a person's dementia is, there can come a time when they will say something inspirational or enlightened, or ask a question such as the one this nurse was asked. (There are of course exceptions to this, when someone may be wordless for many months before they die, but even then can give a smile that lights up the room.) However, if such a question is asked, it is important to take it seriously and not give it an answer that diverts the questioner to some unrelated thought. It may be appropriate to turn the question back onto the person as the nurse realised, and ask how they are feeling right now, so that any preliminary comfort such as a glass or water or a change of pillows can be offered, but the question should then be addressed as honestly as possible, and not ignored.

The Mental Capacity Act (2005) in England and Wales puts forward the significance of planning care in advance, to assist the decision-making of people with dementia in light of their authentic beliefs and principles, while they are still able to do so (Boyle, 2014). Boyle believes a much broader understanding of agency is necessary in the thinking of social science researchers. We need to rely not just on words, but on the many other means that people with dementia depend on to communicate their thoughts and particularly their feelings. (Several approaches are suggested elsewhere in this book – through visual art therapy as well as through sound and embodied somatic movement and gesture (Kontos, 2005).) As quoted in Beausoleil & LeBaron, 2012, "… gestures assist in retrieving words, help to convey ideas, and even play a role in effective problem solving; when physical movement is inhibited, people are notably less capable of these tasks" (Beilock & Goldin-Meadow, 2010; Moore, 2005). In some cases, people with dementia are not offered the physical or psychological space to do this by their spouse, family or main carer. Obviously, an enduring power of attorney may have been selected by the person with dementia ahead of time and authorised to make decisions for their friend or relative. However, challenging though it may be at times for the carer, decisions always need to be checked with the person whose dementia has progressed, and situations such as spouses deciding for their partner because this has been a pattern in their lives, should be avoided (Boyle, 2014).

This respect for agency is, of course, the case for any health professional working with such people at any stage of their lives, but particularly important as they age. As dramatherapists, we structure our individual and group sessions around beginnings and endings, using ritualised activities to mark these moments. We provide grief tables (see Chapter 8) and honour photographs of the dead so that participants can be reminded of the "little deaths" that occur all the time throughout our lives, which can act as a preparation for the main event. Further suggestions for helpful interventions are providing opportunities for touch, mirroring of sound and gesture, and encouraging families to provide treasured objects belonging to the client to touch, feel and consider. Also, activities of scribing for the person and reading back what they have said, and making visual images for the client if they cannot do this themselves, are to be recommended.

Poetry that suggests the mystery of death

For elderly people who have no dementia, and for others who have mild or moderate dementia, inspirational poetry can be a way of leading on to a path where death can be discussed. Some of our best-known poets such as John Donne or William Shakespeare have written about how death acts as a leveller to us as humans: we will all die. There is actually no escape from death. Lines such as Shakespeare's express its inevitability wisely and succinctly:

> Fear no more the heat o'the sun,
> Nor the furious winter's rages;
> Thou thy worldly task hast done,
> Home art gone and ta'en their wages:
> Golden lads and girls all must,
> As chimney-sweepers, come to dust.
>   (Shakespeare, 1876, pp. 4.2.323–328)

Lines such as these connect with the kind of validation therapy that Feil and de Klerk-Rubin (2012) offer in their psychogeriatric approach. Employed artistically and dramatically, these lines can be spoken, rhythmically chanted with the help of percussion instruments, or performed as a dance. Participants can be reminded of their earlier lives as "golden lads and girls", encouraged to talk about their contribution to society through their work or their task as parents and grandparents, as well as reminding each other humorously of why people needed chimney sweeps. It can also bring the discussion around to going "home" when we die, which can in turn lead to a discussion of people's spiritual or religious beliefs. The age group from

70 to 100 years of age is much more likely than many other people to have religious faith.

Poetry and spirit

Rabindranath Tagore, one of the first Indian poets who wrote in English, concerned himself with bereavement and death in a non-denominational and sensitive way. His well-known work, *Gitanjali* (1966) is mainly about love, and in the light of this theme, he writes of the parting that death allots to the relationship between two lovers. He asks the reader to be grateful that the person lived here on earth, telling them that death does not mean the light vanishes, but that the extinguishing of a small lantern means the sun has just risen. Sriprhabar and Srankar (2016) consider his poems as valid on a human level for the "love of the human being, their country, (their) land, for nature and for life itself" (p. 144) and they see Tagore as a spiritual humanist. There are many poems in Gitanjali which are entirely suitable to read to people approaching death.

T. S. Eliot is another poet who brings meaning to the stages of a human life. There is a well-known group of lines in his "Little Gidding", from his Four Quartets, which brings hints of a life journey and the "in-between-ness" (Giesen, 2012) of the twilight years which can be comforting to those with or without a religion. Jungian Helen Luke (2010) points out three gifts that she believes the poet is attributing to old age. Some aspects of these gifts may seem harsh, but there are rewards if one looks deeply. Firstly, very obvious losses of energy and changes in the body senses and strength lead to less clear hearing, sight, smell and taste. Luke refers to the poet's reference to the loss of enchantment, leading to despair. Luke's reading of the poem recalls the despair of developmental psychologist Erikson's (1963) last stage of life, which he equates with "ego integrity versus despair". For Erikson, these losses can somehow diminish the integrity of the self. This binary for a person in that life stage can be somewhat depressing. It might prompt the question, "where am I then on this continuum?" Eliot's gift to the ageing person, on the other hand, is an invitation to live in the here-and-now, and to leave enchantment behind, to the more youthful.

Secondly, Luke views the poet's gift as born out of our frustration, or even rage, against the sense of entitlement of politicians and bureaucrats who hold power in our society. In old age, she says, we need to find a place beyond rage, where we can find joy and laughter. Thirdly, we need to look back at our so-called achievements and find a way to see that what we perceived once as helpful and useful to others in our years of ambition may have been harmful to some others on our way through. There is a place for regret, and the wisdom of old age can see through the lack of maturity we brought to our life earlier on (Luke, 2010).

The following words from T. S. Eliot's Little Gidding give us the sense that we can learn at every stage of our development, gaining wisdom as we go from life stage to life stage, visiting our joys and flaws with new knowledge of the world:

> We shall not cease from exploration
> And the end of all our exploring
> Will be to arrive where we started
> And know the place for the first time.
> Through the unknown, unremembered gate
> When the last of earth left to discover
> Is that which was the beginning;
> At the source of the longest river
> The voice of the hidden waterfall
> And the children in the apple-tree
>
> Not known, because not looked for
> But heard, half-heard, in the stillness
> Between two waves of the sea.
> Quick now, here, now, always—
> A condition of complete simplicity
> (Costing not less than everything)
> And all shall be well and
> All manner of thing shall be well
> When the tongues of flames are in-folded
> Into the crowned knot of fire
> And the fire and the rose are one.
>   (Eliot, 1945, 2002, p. 209)

Eliot's poetry encourages a visit to the "in-between-ness of things" (Giesen, 2012) – the pause between two notes of music, the lacuna in a line of verse and the still moment between breaths. It allows the therapist to slow down to their client's pace and help them remember. This is not just about remembering but re-visiting earlier life stages and acknowledging that humans meet the same experiences over and over again in our lives, but with a certain difference each time because we are older. The poetry can be accompanied by objects and images suggested by the verse, such as pictures of grandchildren and apple trees, waves at the beach, roses and flames. It lends itself to movement and encourages reminiscence.

Dramatherapist Nicky Morris (2011), in her heuristic work with people with dementia, confronts the "paradox of emotions" she experiences, writing her own poetry to unravel the mystery of things while she works with people who have dementia. She writes about the inspiration she draws from Killick, a poet and one-time teacher who has worked tirelessly with creative writing with the aged and ageing, and eschews the medicalised language of the diagnosis. She writes movingly about her ephemeral relationships with her clients and her sense of their cognitive decline: "I face you knowing what you often do not/That you are dying within and the battle is lost". Yet she recognises the unassailable light inside her clients despite their outer disarray: "You may be battered, dishevelled and lost/But you are alive, with spirit and trust" (p. 17). Poetry writing assists her relationally with people with dementia and the counter-transference that is often involved.

My own experience of working with people with dementia has also been made easier by writing about personal counter-transference in verse. For example, on entering the room of a woman just a few years older than myself, my inner response was a sense of "Will this be me one day?"

> She sits, bent double in her chair
> Her head upon her tray
> She's not aware that I am there
> I don't know what to say.
> But then I speak and touch her arm
> I'm in the same life stage.
> My own lost words serve to disarm
> Myself – I'm near her age.
> She straightens up and sits erect
> Greeting me with a smile
> I lose my fear, its cold effect
> That froze me for a while.
> The sparkle in those tired eyes
> The willingness to share
> Bring with them our engaging rise
> Creating – being there.

Although I have not had personal experience of poetry-writing with people in this life stage, I have worked for more than two decades with people who have lived experience of mental illness, some of whom were in their mid-60s. It is a wonderful way of helping clients towards their inner, mysterious wisdom, no matter how difficult their lived experience may be. I have begun by reading a (sometimes famous) poem to them to inspire them and then moved on to writing poetry with them and sharing the results in a group.

For people who are afraid of dying, the words of Henry Scott Holland can be very comforting. The fact that it is written in colloquial language and is very human in its grounded, common-sense attitude, makes it helpful for people who are afraid of death.

> Death is nothing at all.
> I have only slipped away to the next room.
> I am I and you are you.
> Whatever we were to each other,
> That, we still are.

Call me by my old familiar name.
Speak to me in the easy way
which you always used.
Put no difference into your tone.
Wear no forced air of solemnity or sorrow.

Laugh as we always laughed
at the little jokes we enjoyed together.
Play, smile, think of me. Pray for me.
Let my name be ever the household word
that it always was.
Let it be spoken without effect.
Without the trace of a shadow on it.

Life means all that it ever meant.
It is the same that it ever was.
There is absolute unbroken continuity.
Why should I be out of mind
because I am out of sight?

I am but waiting for you.
For an interval.
Somewhere. Very near.
Just around the corner.
All is well.
      (Scott Holland, 1987, no page numbers)

Henry Scott Holland was Canon of Christ Church, Oxford towards the end of the 19th Century. The reader might ask why I chose his poem for this book? I believe he has something important to say to people aged 70 to 100. An advocate of social justice, he had given a eulogy on the death of Edward VII where he brought together the two polarities of fear of the unexplained mystery of death and his belief in continuity. Because elderly people, including those with dementia, feel closer to those who have died (O'Neil & O'Neil, 1990) and because they will be losing friends and acquaintances more frequently than those in other life stages, it is important for them to be given an opportunity to confront death. Even if a resident of a care home does not wish to attend the funeral of someone who has died there, there can still be a morning tea planned where residents can gather to remember the deceased person. The dramatherapist or any other therapist working with these people can bring in a poem such as this one to remind others of the one who has died. Very often, staff will not even want to share the fact of a death with other residents, but a poem like Scott Holland's can help people with dementia think about that person and remember them. An arts therapist or other therapist familiar with the residents is in a privileged position to help with comfort for the bereaved as well as softening fear of people's own death.

The poem can be improvised with people who have mild or moderate dementia, in much the same way as Elspeth's story in Chapter 8. It offers the opportunity of taking imaginary roles, hiding in the "next room", joking and laughter, repeating the names of loved ones who have died and even taking on the role of an angel as Elspeth's story suggested. It goes without saying that any group improvising the poem would need to have established some kind of trust together in order to participate; however, it is feasible in the same way as the death story of Ulu and the breadfruit tree was enacted, also in Chapter 8 (Gersie & King, 1990).

The final poem in this chapter is a more recent one of Mary Oliver's (2017), suggested for people without dementia or with dementia in its mild form. She is an American poet who died in 2019. Many of her poems give a strong message of hope, and her poem "When death comes" is no different. She calls death a little house of darkness and this in itself gives a sense of comfort – it is hardly some cold, columned magisterial hall in which the deceased is frighteningly lonely. It is dark, yes, since it holds a sense of the mysterious. Oliver's own joy in having experienced the joy of the life she would be leaving is palpable. She says that once her life on earth is finished, she has been at her wedding to a sense of wonder, and she was the groom also, as one who embraced the world. When her death comes, she does not want to have negative wonderings and dark thoughts, or to feel as though she was merely a visitor to planet earth.

The idea of having been married to life could still cause some confusion for a person with mild dementia; however, it could bring up suggestions of a marriage partner who has died, and in particular the idea of chasing away the fear of death of the one left behind. It could even be a starting point for a celebration of a deceased partner's life. However, the sheer joy of being both bridegroom and bride, with the Jungian (1991) overtones of animus and anima (see Chapter 1) offers the gift of wholeness to the person who has lived a long life, and an invitation to celebrate their contribution "with open arms" during their time here.

Finally, it is important to note that there are many people, even in our secular society, who find great comfort in their religion, be they Moslem, Jewish, Christian or another. At all levels of society, more literacy in the areas of religion and belief is needed. The 2015 report on religion and belief in British Public Life warns of the risky implications of overlooking these significant elements of human life. The Commission notes the potential for misrepresentation and stereotyping of religion, calling on pedagogical and professional organisations to create belief literacy programs (Butler-Sloss, 2015).

Religious practices that were deeply implanted earlier in life may be of meaningful and reassuring substance for people. This may be the case even when the person has not kept up the affiliation later in life. It is important to have as much understanding as possible of a person's whole life story and not only the beliefs and practices of the later years in order to strike the right note (Kevern, 2015). Naomi Feil (2009), who is Jewish, uses touch, movement and Christian song to help an elderly woman who does not speak, to sing a simple hymn from earlier in her life. She mirrors the woman in the chair with the slightest movement as she encourages her to sing and brings an opportunity for human touch and connection. Mirroring is such a useful technique for assisting people of any age, but especially the elderly. The YouTube video referred to here, working with Gladys Wilson, is a good place to start.

Note

1 Dramatic distancing is a term which covers the method of allowing emotional and psychological problems to be accessed more easily by means of metaphor and symbol (Jones, 2007). A distanced relationship is achieved through projection, for example (see Chapters 3 and 5), to these problems that make them easier to tolerate.

References

Alftberg, A., Ahlstroem, G., Nilsen, P., Behm, L., Benzein, E., Wallerstedt, B., & Rasmussen, B. H. (2018). Conversations about death and dying with older people: An ethnographic study in nursing homes. *Healthcare, 6*(2), 63. https://doi.org/10.3390/healthcare6020063

Beausoleil, E., & LeBaron, M. (2012). What moves us: Dance and neuroscience implications for conflict approaches. *Conflict Resolution Quarterly, 31*(2), 133–158.

Beilock, S. L., & Goldin-Meadow, S. (2010). Gesture changes thought by grounding it in action. *Psychological Science, 21*(11), 1605–1610.

Bell, S. (2019). The spiritual in art therapy at the end of life. In M. M. J. Wood, B. Jacobson, & H. Cridford (Eds.), *The international handbook of art therapy in palliative and bereavement care* (pp. 17–27). Routledge.

Boyle, G. (2014). Recognising the agency of people with dementia. *Disability & Society, 29*(7), 1130–1144. doi: 10.1080/09687599.2014.910108

Butler-Sloss, E. (2015). *Report of the Commission on Religion and Belief in British public life: Living with difference, community, diversity and the common good.* The Woolf Institute.

Byers, A. (1995). Beyond Marks: On working with elderly people with severe memory loss. Inscape Journal of Art Therapy. *British Association of Art Therapists, 1*, 13–18.

Dennes, M., & Gilchrist, S. (2005). *Halfway between everything.* Bonza Street Press.

Dillenbeck, M., & Hammond-Meiers, J. A. (2009). Death and dying: Implications for dance-movement therapy. *American Journal of Dance Therapy, 31*, 95–121.

Eliot, T. S. (1945). *Selected poems.* Harcourt, Brace & Company.

Eliot, T. S. (2002). *Collected poems 1909–1962.* Faber & Faber.

Erikson, E. H. (1963). *Childhood and society.* W. W. Norton.

Feil, N. (1990). Validation therapy helps staff reach confused residents. *Nursing, 16*(12), 33–34.

Feil, N. [Memorybridge]. (2009, May 27). *Gladys Wilson & Naomi Feil* [Video]. YouTube. https://www.youtube.com/watch?v=CrZXz10FcVM

Feil, N. (2012). Validation therapy helps staff reach confused residents. *Nursing*, *16*(12), 33–34.

Feil, N., & de Klerk-Rubin, V. (Eds.). (2012). *The validation breakthrough* (3rd ed.). Health Professions Press.

Gallagher, L. (2013). Creative arts therapies for palliative medicine. *Progress in Palliative Care*, *21*(2), 63–64.

Gersie, A. (1991). *Storymaking in bereavement: Dragons fight in the meadow*. Jessica Kingsley.

Gersie, A., & King, N. (1990). *Storymaking in education and therapy*. Jessica Kingsley.

Giesen, B. (2012). Inbetweenness and ambivalence. In A. Horvath, B. Thomassen, & H. Wydra (Eds.), *Breaking boundaries: Varieties of liminality* (pp. 61–71). Berghahn Books.

Hartley, N., & Payne, M. (2008). *The creative arts in palliative care*. Jessica Kingsley.

Honig, O., Feldman, A., Rinat, S., & Gindi, S. (2019). The chorus of angels, the ripple of water and the weight of stone: Art therapy and art work which cradle both family carers and their relative with dementia. In M. M. J. Wood, B. Jacobson, & H. Cridford (Eds.), *The international handbook of art therapy in palliative and bereavement care* (pp. 161–180). Routledge International.

Jones, P. (2007). *Drama as therapy: Theory, practice and research* (2nd ed.). Routledge.

Jung, C. J. (1991). *The structure and dynamics of the psyche* (2nd ed.). Princeton University Press.

Kevern, P. (2015). The spirituality of people with late-stage dementia: A review of the research literature, a critical analysis and some implications for person-centred spirituality and dementia care. *Mental Health, Religion and Culture*, *18*(9), 765–776.

Kohn, L. (1993). Validating current validation therapy. (Letter to the Editor). *Journal of Gerontological Nursing*, *19*(11), 6.

Kontos, P. (2005). Embodied selfhood in Alzheimer's disease: Rethinking person-centred care. *Dementia*, *4*(4), 553–570.

Kübler-Ross, E. (1969). *On death and dying*. MacMillan Publishing Company Inc.

Luke, H. (2010). *Old age*. Lindisfarne Books.

Mannix, K. (2017). *With the end in mind*. William Collins.

Mental Capacity Act. UK Public General Acts. (2005). https://www.legislation.gov.uk/ukpga/2005/9/contents

Moore, C.-L. (2005). *Movement and making decisions: The body-mind connection in the workplace*. Dance and Movement Press.

Morris, N. (2011). Unspoken depths: Dramatherapy and dementia. *Dramatherapy*, *33*(3), 144–157.

Oliver, M. (2017). *Devotions*. Penguin Random House LLC.

O'Neil, G., & O'Neil, G. (1990). *The human life*. Mercury Press.

Redhouse, R. (2015). Life story: Meaning making through dramatherapy in a palliative care context. *Dramatherapy*, *36*(2–3), 66–80.

Salmon, D. (2001). Music therapy as psychospiritual process in palliative care. *Journal of Palliative Care*, *17*, 142–146.

Scott-Holland, H. (1987). *Death is nothing at all*. Souvenir Press Ltd.

Shakespeare, W. (1876). *The dramatic works of William Shakespeare* (T. Campbell, Ed.). George Routledge & Sons.

Small, N., Froggatt, K., & Downs, M. (2007). *Living and dying with dementia: Dialogues about palliative care*. Oxford University Press.

Sriprhabar, M., & Srankar, G. (2016). Themes of adore and bereavement in Tagore's Gitanjali – A study. *International Journal of English Literature and Culture*, *4*(8), 142–145.

Tagore, R. (1966). *Gitanjali*. Macmillan India, Ltd.

The, A-M. (2008). *In death's waiting room: Living and dying with dementia in a multi-cultural society*. Amsterdam University Press.

Warth, M., Keßler, J., Hillecke, T. K., & Bardenheuer, H. J. (2015). Music therapy in palliative care. *Deutsches Ärzteblatt International*, *112*, 788–794.

Warth, M., Koenig, J., Keßler, J., Wormit, A. F., Hillecke, T. K., & Bardenheuer, H. J. (2014). Musiktherapie in der palliativmedizinischen Versorgung: Gegenwärtiger Stand und aktuelle Entwicklungen. *Musiktherapeutische Umschau*, *35*, 261–274.

Wilks, R., & Byers, A. (1992). Art therapy with elderly people in statutory care. In A. Gilroy, & D. Waller (Eds.), *Art therapy, a handbook* (pp. 90–104). Open University Press.

Chapter 10

Assessment and evaluation

In the previous chapter, the end of life was considered, together with various ways in which people with dementia could be offered opportunities to prepare for this event. Bearing in mind that in facilities for the elderly so little mention is made of death until a person reaches the stage of palliative care, it is important to engage them in a celebration of their life together with possibilities of conscious awareness of its culmination. Calling on literature and poetry, together with some of the questions that people with dementia and their families ask, as well as some of the other questions which hang in the air unasked in old age, suggestions of artistic ways to attend to these questions were put forward during my research. These activities contribute to people's quality of life (QoL). The present chapter describes three assessment tools which help the therapist measure aspects of QoL, and explains how to use them. One is a quantitative scale designed directly to investigate 13 aspects of QoL, a second has creative implications for aspects of QoL as indicated by people with dementia themselves (Alzheimer's Society, 2010; Moyle et al., 2011) and the third is a dramatherapy-based tool suitable for all life stages.

Dramatherapist and psychologist Caroline Miller (2014), writing about the book she edited on assessment in the arts therapies, assembled case studies and models, showing how therapists can easily include versatile measurement in their practices. She finds that this approach can promote a common understanding about the goals of therapy and shed light on the methods, techniques and models of therapy that can help the client most. She believes that formalising process in a client-centred way is to be encouraged, and doing so gives direction to both client and therapist about the goals and outcomes of the therapy they are both involved in (Miller, 2014). It can also facilitate an alignment with the aims and mission statements of the organisations which employ them.

In Chapter 4, a research project was described where the improvement of QoL of people with dementia who were offered dramatherapy was investigated. For the purposes of this research, measures to assess QoL were selected. Two of these were not tested through Statistical Package for the Social Sciences (SPSS) software. Both were assessment tools with a creative arts component.

DOI: 10.4324/9781003186328-10

Quality of life in Alzheimer's disease

With regard to the quantitative measure, a literature search for evidence-based QoL scales was made as a means of comparison and to assess ways in which dramatherapy adds value to clients' lives. A mixed method approach was considered an optimum procedure for conducting the study and to triangulate quantitative results with qualitative outcomes. QoL is a complex area and authors like Wendy Moyle see this aspect of dementia care as having been largely ignored and worthy of much greater examination (Moyle et al., 2007). Since co-writing about this deficit in 2007, she and her colleagues have relied upon the excellent validity and reliability elements of the quality of life, Alzheimer's disease scale (QoL-AD) (Logsdon et al., 1999, 2002) on at least three occasions in their research. Moyle et al. (2007) recommend it, among other characteristics, for its absence of emphasis on pathology. She and her colleagues have done this with a view to evaluating topics strictly associated with the quality of people's lives, comparing self-report and proxy accounts (Moyle et al., 2011). They conclude that the QoL-AD scale is successful in representing the viewpoints of the research cohort who have dementia. This comparative research by Moyle and her colleagues has acted as a base to superimpose an algorithm from another author allowing for five further specific qualities added to the scale (Welch & Comans, 2019) and to investigate these qualities more thoroughly, based on the QoL-AD (Comans et al., 2018).

The QoL-AD was selected in the study for its strengths, since it gives agency to people with dementia to assess their own QoL and offers them an opportunity of freedom from the "disease narrative" emphasised by some other QoL measures. The scale requires a carer or family member to answer identical questions alongside each participant, but the scoring is weighted in favour of the person with dementia. A QoL-AD participant score is produced by doubling it and adding the caregiver's score, whereupon the sum is divided by three to arrive at a composite score which gives the person with dementia the heavier rating (Logsdon et al., 1999).

Two groups of participants, the dramatherapy group and the one doing usual activities, were measured at baseline (T1) and after completing 16 sessions (T2). The scale itself (Logsdon, 1996) contains questions which range from enquiries about physical health and energy levels, through mood, living situation and relationships. It covers self-management, ability to undertake various activities, finances and life as a whole. These questions are in general appropriate for people living in the community or in aged care facilities, although the question about finance is less appropriate. Such questions would for the most part need to be dealt with by a power of attorney, especially once the person was in a care home. Little difficulty was experienced by participants in answering the questions using the four alternative responses: poor, fair, good or excellent. The replies of people with dementia tended to be more positive than those of the family members or carers for people living in the community like the people in this study (Jaaniste, 2013). QoL scores for the cohort described in this book may be seen in Figure 4.1, at the end of Chapter 4.

In the study, there were only 13 volunteers out of 80 possible participants identified at the start of the program who went on to complete all 16 sessions and all final assessments. The volunteers came from a database provided by the organisation which ran both centres where the investigation was made. As a result of the small size of the cohorts, the potential of the study in being able to identify the change in the QoL-AD scores was compromised by the small sample size. Secondly, the modest number involved in the project meant there was a limited ability to match participants on factors such as baseline QoL, diagnosis, gender and age (Jaaniste et al., 2015).

In comparing the two groups, it can be observed from Figure 4.1 (p. 44 in Chapter 4) that there was a difference between the two groups at the end point of the project (T2) and the dramatherapy group's average score increased from T1 to T2 while the film group's average score decreased from T1 to T2. It is likely that with a larger sample size, the results may have been statistically significant and the matter certainly warrants further investigation, which is why I am recommending it here.

Creative-Expressive Abilities Assessment (CEAA)

As noted in Chapter 4, my research was informed by the views expressed by people with dementia when they were assisted to name the essential attributes of QoL with the help of talking mats and storyboards (Jaaniste et al., 2015). The full list of these attributes is given here and stated in order of importance: relationships, environment, physical health, sense of humour, independence, ability to communicate, sense of personal identity, ability to engage in activities, ability to practise faith or religion and ability to be treated fairly (Alzheimer's Society, 2010, pp. 17–22).

These qualities still seem to me to depend on the opportunities afforded to people with dementia through creative activity which improve QoL in dramatherapy sessions. CEAA (Gottlieb-Tanaka et al., 2016) differs somewhat from those mentioned above. These are: memory, attention, language, psychosocial, reasoning/problem-solving, emotions and culture. Although not defined as essential by people with dementia, they share aspects of the qualities stated in the paragraph above, and have shown improvement when older people with dementia have participated in creative activity programs (Verity & Lee, 2011). The results of the CEAA assessment in my study identified the average scores of all participants in these areas for each session – all important areas of awareness in any consideration of QoL. The CEAA tool was not used in the control group, as participants were mainly seated spectators, watching films, with little or no time for creative discussion of the movies afterwards (Jaaniste, 2016). When using this assessment tool for groups, it may be helpful to bring together all the individual scores for each session and put the data into graph form for each attribute.

These observations using the CEAA tool are not as precise as the statistically examined quantitative research where participants gave their own personal assessments. However, they provide a very useful guide, from shared indications observed by the three health professionals and two art therapy students assisting the group, as to what actually changed in the participants' QoL. There is no specific requirement for a certain number of observers to make observations. In McAdam's (2012) investigation into an ongoing art therapy experience to establish well-being in participants, the assessment was made with one observer present and two others who viewed video of the sessions. Observers in my study provided clues after each session as to why change occurred during the 16 weeks of dramatherapy sessions. Their brief was to observe each of the participants carefully and to assess to what extent they fulfilled each attribute, i.e. M2: Did the participant remember a song, story or joke during the session? They looked for change in verbal expression, body language and engagement. If there was a significant difference of opinion in the observer group, this was discussed before allotting an agreed score. In almost all cases, except for the section on cultural attributes, there was an overall average improvement in QoL of the dramatherapy group participants.

The authors Gottlieb-Tanaka et al. (2016) were interested in gerontology and dementia and wanted to enable the kind of data harvesting that would provide answers to their questions about the effectiveness and character of multiple forms of creative–expressive work for seniors. They also wanted to know if there were variances in the program benefits for people with different levels of dementia.

The CEAA was designed with 25 core items along with two optional writing items, which are there for use in programs which offer some kind of creative writing involvement. This option was useful in Ben's case, since he was much more comfortable with writing and script than with the drawing and painting activities offered. A statistical analysis of the data from the final 25-item CEAA showed it to have good internal consistency, with a Cronbach's alpha score $= 0.86$, thereby indicating that all of the items are sensitive to the same general underlying construct. Across the individual items, the Cohen's κ scores ranged from a low of 0.20 to a high of 0.75. An analysis of the total scores, defined as the sum of all item scores across the 25-item CEAA, produced a Cramér's V score of 0.825 (Cramér, 1999) and a contingency coefficient of 0.975 (Gottlieb-Tanaka et al., 2016).

There are five possible scores for each participant's expressive ability in each area: 0 = no observation; 1 = never observed; 2 = rarely observed; 3 = sometimes observed; and 4 = always or nearly always observed. Those rating the abilities familiarised themselves with the rating method in advance of the group sessions. The individual scores for each of the items can be averaged for a group as well as understood as stand-alone scores. Scores were recorded and provided useful information about group average declines and improvements.

Memory

This domain has three main items. Memory is evidenced by talking about or improvising incidents which occurred in the recent or more distant past (M1), remembering songs, stories or jokes (M2), and/or adding additional information to a discussion or performance (M3).

Reminiscence showed a decline to an average of 2 (rarely observed) for the group in the early part of the 16 sessions and then a steady rise to 3 (sometimes observed) where the instances of memory showed a sharp improvement in Session 7, with memories of grief and loss, stimulated by the story of "Ulu and the breadfruit tree" (Gersie & King, 1990). It dropped to 2 again in Session 9, just after the two-week break, probably because participants needed to get used to meeting one another again. Group rate of remembering went up to 3.5 in Session 11 when Leanne enacted her anger towards the teacher who had emotionally abused her, as her work stimulated multiple memories in others.

Attention

This attribute is confined to a singular item (A4) which refers to the duration of time participants are able to apply their attention to the drama, visual art or singing during an activity, or to the conversation in a period of reflection.

Average attention in the group began at 3 at the beginning of the group and dropped in Session 2, to an average score of 2. Once again, the group needed to get to know and trust one another initially and this may explain the decline in score. After the march to Parliament House in Session 4, the score rose in Session 5 and stayed steadily there until the program ended in Session 16. It was hypothesised that participants' memory had improved with stimulation, especially as Session 4 was arousing and active and Session 5 presented them with the opportunity for active somatic work culminating in a dance-movement exercise.

Language

This third area of language comprises eight items. The first two items are rated on the participant's ability to write (L5) or speak (L6) complete words and full sentences which transfer a useful message. Item L7 asks for a rating of body language which relates to simultaneously spoken words.

Items L8 and L9 refer to writing or speaking humorously, to wit or teasing, or for appreciating humour in a situation. Item L10 relates to a narrative of real situations occurring in a participant's life, or situations they have invented. Item L11 is concerned with rhythmic body language or facial expressions used by participants when appreciating music and L12 to singing along or simultaneously moving their lips.

Language scores did not shift greatly. They started at about 2.8 and moved to an end point of about 3.5. All participants but one shared English as a first language, and the level of education was higher than in the control group doing usual activities. It is postulated that the high score in Session 16 might be because of the addition of more singing than usual and a celebratory atmosphere.

Psychosocial

The psychological and social aspects of participant expression involve eye contact, voicing and expression of feeling when storytelling or narrating an anecdote (P13), singing (P14) or performing (P15). The hearers' or viewers' eye contact, affect and gestures relay information about the levels of heed they pay to the participant's narration or performance.

Item P16 rates the attention to others' contributions; a thoughtful comment would attract a higher score and a one-word answer a lower score. Item P27 relates mainly to the participant's elucidation of their own or their family's accomplishments and future plans. Grooming (P18) refers to a participant's dress and interest in their own appearance.

Once again, there was a small improvement in the psychosocial level from Sessions 1 to 16, from approximately 2.7 to 3.2. Confidence peaked at Session 4, where the protest improvisation took place, and that score was very much lifted by Neil, who was marked at 4 on every item in this domain except for P14. There was increased interest in the activities and productions of others as the time went on, showing greater sociability,

Reasoning/problem solving

In this domain, the kinds of insights shown are those which, for item R19, comment on the dramatic or other artistic performance (e.g. where someone should stand at a certain time [and/or] the placement or arrangement of objects in space). For item R20, rating is based on personal choices made in the process of performance or conversation/reflection.

Over the 16 sessions, the group insight and reasoning ability started at just over 2, declining to 1.8 in Session 3. There was also a decline in that session in the memory and psychosocial areas. All of this suggests a slump in Session 3 which coincided with the beginning of the "storming" period referred to elsewhere which continued in Session 4 (see Chapter 5). However, a reading of the scores shows a much greater autonomy in reasoning and decision-making towards the end of the period, when Leanne was dealing finally with her childhood issue and participants were taking responsibility for finding solutions and making decisions. Between Sessions 14 and 16, the score rose from 2.5 to 3.5.

Emotions

Elsewhere in this book, I have referred to a preference for the word "feelings" rather than "emotions" because the latter refers more accurately to the intelligent/conscious genre of emotion. Regarding this complex area of feeling life, item E21 rates as opening the eyes widely, nodding, frowning or smiling by a participant. E22 refers to these kinds of responses as a result of looking at a painting or photograph, observing a drama performance or another's roleplay. Body language and rhythmic movement as well as conversation about the music the participant is hearing or singing constitute a rating for E23. Item E24 refers to the enthusiasm or interest the participant conveys when relating incidents or stories of their life.

The expression of feeling was quite flat for the first three sessions and then began to improve until it reached its first peak in Session 5 where some dance-movement work was achieved, and participants planted seeds. This improvement began in Session 4, with the protest march. It is possible that the strong emotions expressed in Session 4 were connected with the simultaneous improvement in memory, above. Progress then remained level until Session 12 when it began to rise to 3.5 at Session 15. The mood in that session was energised and inspired by vicarious group enthusiasm where the participants helped Leanne to "dismiss" Mrs. L from the "playground". The scores showed a clear lift in expression of mood and feeling.

Culture: Spirituality, religion, traditions, customs

This section refers to religious belief and views on the supernatural, cultural mores and ritual. C25 concerns the occasions when a participant shares deep thoughts or feelings from the heart in a meaningful way, verbally or through performance or movement. Tone of voice is considered in observation as well as cultural background. C26 applies to philosophical or moral advice or lessons about life. It can also touch on regrets or situations still to be resolved. C27 concerns questions about religion and the existence of God, reward for good deeds and the good/evil binary.

This attribute is the only one where scores show an overall decline. It is understandable that early sessions did not provide examples of wisdom or spiritual input, as participants were getting to know one another. Session 6 (2.5) is the first occasion when the average score rose; Leanne and Neil both had wise and deep thoughts about child abuse and lack of connection between some fathers and their children. Once again, in Session 9 (2.6), life and death in the era of World War I was discussed. Parental values were performed and expressed verbally, when children were allowed in the surf when parents were not present. In the next session, scores plummeted to 1.4 and the mood was very flat. It is likely that the low 1.7 score of the ending of dramatherapy sessions left participants feeling sad at Session 16 (Jaaniste, 2013). The most recent (Gottlieb-Tanaka et al., 2016) version of the Creative Expressive Abilities Assessment is available from the internet address in the reference section.

Discussion of the CEAA

One of the most significant reasons for choosing this assessment tool was its facility to use with groups as well as individuals. The change in scores for memory and emotion shows that stimulation, often resulting in strong feelings, assists with memory. This was not a longitudinal study; however, it is likely that improvements and new-found interests were transferable to other areas of participants' lives. In the community, where these participants were living, there were likely to have been some changes, and these have been reported anecdotally by carers. After more than 12 months, Leanne's husband/carer reported the absence of any reference to the difficult issue of her troublesome teacher, a memory which he and others had referred to as "obsessive". He also acknowledged a new enjoyable playfulness in his interactions with her, especially at bedtimes, which had previously been problematic for them both. We observed a cross-fertilisation of interests and a depth of immersion in art works and drama that showed what could be achieved if participants were to continue with this work. Socially, this was demonstrated through a camaraderie which alleviated the loneliness that often arises from receiving the diagnosis. Most participants took their art works home, enabling others to realise that people with dementia do not just "eat the paint" (McAdam, 2012, p. 381)!

Jones' (1996) Adaptation of Scale of Dramatic Involvement (JASDI)

This JASDI scale (Jaaniste, 2013) which was originally the Sutton-Smith Lazier Scale of Dramatic Involvement (Sutton-Smith, 1981), was initially designed to measure drama sessions. Jones (1996) modified it for use by dramatherapists, and it was re-adapted for the research project described in this book. The scale has been simplified, presenting the scoring system as percentages of involvement in the dramatherapy by participants.

Table 10.1 gives the opportunity for client attributes to be expressed as percentages. This method has been selected because the original scale required selecting one, two, three, four or five according to the extent to which an attribute was observed. In the JASDI version, each part is thus given a value

Table 10.1 Jones's Adaption of Sutton-Smith, Lazier, Scale of Dramatic Involvement

Client ID	Session	Focus within activity as a whole behaviours	Focus with "as if"	Completion	Use of imaginary objects – pretended objects	Use of imaginary objects – disengage when end	Use of imaginary objects – other's objects	Elaboration – initiate own ideas	Elaboration – engage with others' elaboration	Use of space	Facial expression	Body movement – using own body	Body movement – understanding other's bodies	Vocal expression	Social relationships	Attributes compilation (ave. of attributes)
										Client attributes – expressed on a percentage scale						
Ben	2	38	12	16	0	0	12	16	0	16	16	16	16	16	16	14
Ben	16	63	63	50	100	100	88	50	75	50	50	50	50	50	50	64
David	2	63	38	50	100	100	12	50	0	50	16	50	50	50	16	46
David	11	88	88	83	100	100	63	50	75	50	83	83	50	50	50	72

in the final score on the chart. The original adapted scale (Jones, 1996) can be found above. It was re-adjusted by taking a simple assessment requiring only yes/no answers and adapting them in percentage form to produce attributes encompassing a varying number of points. An example of this, an attribute which had three points might be as follows:

Attribute: Completion of tasks
Points: Completes all tasks; Completes some tasks; Completes no tasks
Scores are given for a three-point attribute as follows:
Completes all tasks: (67–100%) 83
Completes some tasks: (34–66%) 50
Completes no tasks: (0–33%) 16

In my study, two sessions – one earlier and one later in the programme – were focused on for each of two participants in order to discuss changes in capacities such as body movement, use of space and elaboration of action. I wanted to see in which ways and how much these elements of their expression had changed over the program. I watched the video of the sessions in order to make assessments. Ben and David were selected for this measurement process. They were chosen on the basis that they had begun the program quite static in their movements. In the early session with a climate theme, for example, Session 2, most of the participants were walking around, improvising their movements as if in various types of weather. In this session, there was little body movement in either Ben or David's case; improvisation and interaction with others were missing when the "weather" changed from cold to warm to wind and showers. Both stood still, watching while others created a snowman in improvisation, despite staff and students' endeavours to help them to join in. Their facial expressions were blank, even though they were both able to engage in conversation. There was a snowball fight which neither participant engaged in, although they both took art materials and Ben wrote, yet neither showed any facial expression. I chose this session as the first of two for each of them in making a comparison over the whole program. It can be observed from the graph that Ben could not improvise an imaginary object such as putting up an umbrella, or engage with others' improvisations even if approached – he scored zero in each case. David had a low score (12) for improvising imaginary objects, such as finding ways to help build a snowman, and shared with Ben a zero score for engaging with others' dramatic expressions.

The two later chosen sessions were different in each case. David's lifelong occupation had been as a solicitor sitting behind a desk or else in court all his working life; it was difficult for him to use his body expressively. In Session 11, there was dressing up and concrete material for him to use in his somatic movement and taking advantage of the space, he showed far more somatic and facial expression. The topic was "Dealing with difficult people" and he was involved in two improvisations, the first where he needed to deal with a con-man in role and the second which was a lived experience of a rebellious lad at school, mentioned in Chapter 8. In this session also, he was involved with an improvised bullfight, and he additionally dressed and moved around as a gay man. His score for pretending to use an object had risen to 63 and engaging with others' work had improved to 75.

These improvements in David's scores bear out Kontos' (2012) view that the embodied self in dementia "discloses social and cultural movements and physical cues that derive from the internalisation of a sociocultural environment through one's primary socialisation" (p. 29). She bases her ideas in this regard upon both Merleau-Ponty's (1962) and Bourdieu's (1977) views that suggest a new way of perceiving, promoting an approach to a selfhood that takes into account the pre-reflective body and the strength of its natural expression. In other words, we consider the connected motor and tactile elements of our body and the totality of its movements that come from early socialisation and cultural input. The power of this concept has significant implications for how we read and observe the body language of people with dementia, especially those experiencing its final stages. Ben was approaching this last stage, with its acute difficulties in word retention.

The concluding chapter of this book refers once again to this phenomenon, as it brings together some of the questions and approaches suggested in the book, in offering the arts therapies, and in particular dramatherapy, to this population experiencing every stage of dementia.

References

Alzheimer's Society. (2010). *My name is not dementia: People with dementia discuss quality of life indicators*. Author.

Bourdieu, P. (1977). *Outline of a theory of practice* (R. Nice, Trans.). Cambridge University Press.

Comans, T. A., Nguyen, K.-H., Mulhern, B., Corlis, M., Li, L., Welch, A., Currle, S. E., Rowen, D., Moyle, W., Kularatna, S., & Ratcliffe, J. (2018). Developing a dementia-specific, preference-based quality of life measure (AD-5D) in Australia: A validation study protocol. *British Medical Journal Open, 8*, Article e018996. doi:10.1136/bmjopen-2017-018996

Cramér, H. (1999). *Mathematical methods of statistics*. Princeton University Press.

Gersie, A., & King, N. (1990). *Storymaking in education and therapy*. Jessica Kingsley.

Gottlieb-Tanaka, D., Lee, H., & Graf, P. (2016). *Creative Expressive Abilities Assessment user guide*. ArtScience Press. Retrieved July 7, 2021, from http://www.dementia-activities.com/product_CEAA_Tool.html#:~:text=The%20Creative%2D Expressive%20Abilities%20Assessment,participated%20in%20creative%20 activity%20programs

Jaaniste, E. J. (2013). *Pulled through a hedge backwards: Improving the quality of life of people with dementia through dramatherapy* [Unpublished PhD Thesis]. University of Western Sydney.

Jaaniste, J. (2016). The role of dramatherapy in improving quality of life. *Australian Journal of Dementia Care, 5*(2), 24–26.

Jaaniste, J., Linnell, S., Ollerton, S., & Slewa-Younan, R. L. (2015). Dramatherapy with elders with dementia – Does it improve quality of life? *The Arts in Psychotherapy*, *43*, 40–48.

Jones, P. (2006). *Drama as therapy: Theatre as living*. Routledge.

Kontos, P. (2012). Rethinking sociability in long-term care: An embodied dimension of selfhood. *Dementia*, *11*(3), 329–346.

Logsdon, R. (1996). *Quality of Life Alzheimer's Disease*. Author. Retrieved June 26, 2021, from https://www.cogsclub.org.uk/professionals/files/QOL-AD.pdf

Logsdon, R., Gibbons, L., McCurry, S., & Teri, L. (1999). Quality of life in Alzheimer's disease: Patient and caregiver reports. *Journal of Mental Health & Ageing*, *5*, 21–32.

Logsdon, R. G., Gibbons, L. E., McCurry, S. M., & Teri, L. (2002). Assessing quality of life in older adults with cognitive impairment. *Psychosomatic Medicine*, *64*, 510–519.

McAdam, J. G. (2012). *The relationship between art and wellbeing in individuals living with dementia* [Unpublished PhD Thesis]. Victoria University.

Merleau-Ponty, M. (1962). *Phenomenology of perception* (C. Smith, Trans.). Routledge & Kegan Paul.

Miller, C. (2014). (Ed.). *Assessment and outcomes in the arts therapies*. Jessica Kingsley.

Moyle, W., McAllister, M., Venturato, L., & Adams, T. (2007). Quality of life & dementia. *Dementia*, *6*(2), 175–191.

Moyle, W., Murfield, J. E., Griffiths, S. G., & Venturato, L. (2011). Assessing quality of life of older people with dementia: A comparison of quantitative self-report and proxy accounts. *Journal of Advanced Nursing*, *68*(10), 2237–2246.

Sutton-Smith, B. (1981). Sutton Smith-Lazier scale of dramatic involvement. In G. Schattner & R. Courtney (Eds.), *Drama in therapy* (Vol. 1). Drama Book Specialists.

Verity, J., & Lee, H. (2011). Reigniting the human spirit. In H. Lee, & T. Adams (Eds.), *Creative approaches in dementia care* (pp. 16–31). Palgrave Macmillan.

Welch, A., & Comans, T. (2019). Confirmatory analysis of a health state classification system for people living with dementia: A qualitative approach. *Journal of Health Services Research & Policy*, *24*(4), 256–265.

Chapter 11

Conclusion

As this book draws to a close, it seems significant to try to bring some of the threads together for an ending that looks to the future of offering dramatherapy in working with the creativity of people with dementia. However, this drawing-together does not preclude the presence of some final questions which remain. Whether or not we are dramatherapists, we are therapist-researchers who question how people with dementia benefit from the arts, and from the arts therapies in particular.

David Whyte (2016) talks about a youthful sense we are meant to grow into once we are 70 or 80 as we journey to life's end. He attributes to it a quality of surprise and unfolding discovery that belongs to our humanness, together with what will be gifted onward for others – the image and shape of our absence. In this conclusion, I ask myself whether this statement can be true of our fellow human beings who have dementia. This is one of the deep questions I am left with as I reflect on the sense of wonder and aware contemplation in many of the people who have given permission for me to record their thoughts and feelings within its pages.

Whyte is referring to our generativity (intergenerational sensitivity) – a concept for which Tornstam's (1997) research uncovered a new level: a "gerotranscendence". This attribute that people report on as they approach the later stages of life is related to an understanding of time that differs entirely from how they have seen it in previous life stages. His investigative interviews with elders reveal that for some, the past might be present in a way whereby they are *re-experiencing* it while at the same time living the actual moment of describing it. These elders do not have dementia, but their idea of yesterday has melded into today. Others report an almost daily re-visiting of their childhood, one woman saying she now "dares" to go there. Time seems to collapse in on itself, with ancestors feeling closer to the person, and past history not seeming very far away from their present experience. This is borne out by Tornstam's interviewees: ordinary language was inadequate to express these feelings and for one man, art, drama and music could bring him to an awareness he was not able to attain through language. For others, celebrations and other such excitements belonged to earlier life stages and

DOI: 10.4324/9781003186328-11

had been replaced by small and more so-called ordinary experiences, often connected with nature.

These investigative approaches into late life stages from Chapter 1 highlight a connection with the feeling intelligence that was introduced in Chapter 5 – a refined ability involving memory and awareness. Even in the presence of cognitive disintegration in dementia, Tornstam's research flags another feature of later life stages, shared by Joan Erikson (1997) as a normal feature of ageing. What is revealed by both these thinkers is knowledge that is very useful to therapists working artistically with people with dementia. It informs us that the ability to take part in projective exercises and role-play can be a natural way of revisiting some of those earlier memories which are closer to the reality of older people than they were earlier in life. It justifies the approach taken in the project described in these pages that people with dementia are often happy to explore their past, share stories of their lives and find meaning in their memories.

Early in the book, the diagnosis of several types of dementia was discussed and some aspects often referred to as symptoms were compared with normal changes that occur in later life stages anyway. Naturally, many of these symptoms, such as forgetfulness, social withdrawal and feeling closer to those who have died can be experienced in a more acute sense by someone who has dementia. However, it is not helpful to interpret normal developmental signs as symptoms of disease. The thoughts and feelings of the people in the program, in the session that followed in Chapter 2, showed that not everyone's attitude to their dementia diagnosis is the same, and neither is the way they manage it. Participants showed their pleasure in movement and song, as they were reminded of the seeds they had planted in their lives so far. Opportunities for growth and resilience were still there, and the metaphor of growth lent authenticity to their identities as continuously developing human beings.

Chapter 3 explored the aims and holistic nature of dramatherapy and the significance of body, mind and spirit when working therapeutically with elders and people with dementia in particular. Connected with holism is the art of play, which is recommended for people of all ages, but particularly for people with dementia. There are questions related to this: does this kind of activity infantilise these participants? Disinhibition, which is a symptom of dementia, discussed earlier in the book, can lead to anxiety on the part of managers, carers and families. It can be disturbing to watch a loved one, for example, start to undress in an inappropriate setting. There might be times when their client or loved person embarrasses themselves or others with their behaviour. Families and others also have questions about the respect they quite rightly feel is due to their client or relative and may be anxious about infantilisation of elders. But there is a substantial difference between offering play and putting a bow in an elder's hair and calling them "love" rather than by their name, which I would suggest is infantilising them. A carer may not recognise that to be disinhibited helps the person to play and be spontaneous, in a way that someone more guarded or circumspect might not wish to. It is up to the individual dramatherapist or any therapist offering artistic expression to show how a combination of treating the client with humanity and allowing them to play can lift mood, bring humour and assist with socialisation.

In Chapter 6, the concept of quality of life (QoL) was discussed along with the change in Australia from this quality-based model of dementia care to the approach of the Royal Commission into Aged Care Quality and Safety (2019), where safety seems to be the main topic of concern. I have referred earlier to the fact that the word "life" has not been mentioned in connection with "quality". This discussion was in the context of artificial intelligence (AI) and its effect on people with dementia. Safety must of course be seriously considered, but the QoL of such people is highly dependent on the delivery of person-centred care, investing their lives with quality. A person-centred approach is relational, depending as it does on interpersonal contact, maintaining relationships where possible and championing dignity and respect at the same time. The introduction of AI in areas where human-to-human conversation and touch still belong should always include major questions about how we offer people dignity and respect alongside the technology. Surely, if we are to fulfil the requirements of quality care that respects their life, their history and their identity, we need to use AI with discernment and clear-eyed awareness of what it may be replacing.

The chapter on AI is followed by another on client responses to trauma, and how to deal with post-traumatic stress disorder (PTSD) in people who have dementia. The decision to place these two chapters next to each other was a deliberate one. Our work with embodiment as therapists – in drama or any clinical profession – can help the person with dementia in areas that are unlikely to be offered to them by means of AI. I hope for the reader following Leanne's progress throughout 16 sessions of dramatherapy, for example, it has been made clear that her willingness to engage in active play brought her eventually to a state of peace about her childhood memory of not being allowed to do so as a nine-year-old. This kind of play is not possible, to my knowledge, with technology or with robots. Leanne was not only assisted by the enjoyment of the play she threw herself into, but by the active involvement of others in the games. Her embodiment of imaginary scenarios in Developmental Transformations (Johnson, 2009), collaboration in a dance movement exercise, and other games encouraged her body to tell her reflective mind it could forget about the traumatic experience (van der Kolk, 2015). For other participants, there were less dramatic yet useful opportunities to release themselves of their own traumatic responses through embodiment witnessed and reflected upon in sessions.

The question of spirituality and religious affiliation in dementia care is one which has been mentioned throughout, belonging as it does to QoL and person-centred care. In 2014, Agli et al. examined 51 articles for a systematic review on this topic (Agli et al., 2014). Out of 51 papers researching affiliation and whether it could be influential in health maintenance or recovering from illness, 11 articles were chosen for investigation. Cognitive ability, coping strategies, and QoL in people with dementia were examined. The majority showed that people's spiritual or religious faith in daily life enabled them to develop the means to find acceptance for their dementia, hold onto their relationships, live hopefully and meaningfully and thereby improve their quality of life.

Reviews of this kind assist the dramatherapist and others to look out for such affiliations, signs and questions of transpersonal belief. In an overwhelmingly secular Western society, it is easy to forget that elders have sometimes had a lifetime of drawing on such sources and they can be a positive force for good in their lives. It is always helpful for therapists to carry, along with other concrete objects useful for projective work, some that are symbolic of their clients' faiths, preferably belonging to diverse religions. When I was working with Khmer people in a mental health setting some years ago, it was important to bring objects reminiscent of their religion – among them a tiny model of Ankar Wat temple and a sounding bowl – as well as Christian symbols for those who had no Buddhist affiliations.

In Chapter 8, questions about grief and loss were discussed. I believe it is important to ask a further question here about whether any gains (rather than losses) exist, although not widely reported in the literature, among people who have dementia. Offering dramatherapy, one of these gains could be considered the release of what Gersie calls "grief (kept) under tight control" (1991, p. 232). Neil's memory of his mother and expression of grief about her death came from the everyday scent of fruit. This ordinary occurrence shows that we don't always need historic reminiscence objects like bus tickets or traditional egg timers to bring grief to the fore when working with elders. The gains that were made in that interaction were manifold. Neil found that taking a role of his very young self in his Mum's kitchen and being chased around the table by Leanne in her role left him with a strong sense of her ability to have fun. Her tolerance of his mischief in pinching pieces of apple she was preparing supported him in the role of his childhood self. It provided him with a confirmation of his own maturity in realising that indeed he couldn't have his Mum forever, but he did have the ability to re-visit his loving memories of her. It gave Leanne a playful role that she could just manage to hold, helping Neil in his re-enactment of a youthful memory. The reader may have other questions, or indeed answers, about gains as opposed to losses for the person with dementia in the later stages of life.

The matter of how to approach death is one we all face as human beings, and there are serious questions about abandoning conversations about death with ageing people, as discussed in Chapter 9. Because death is a mystery and no one comes back to tell us what happens next, there are obviously many questions, but this does not mean leaving the biggest ending of all without reflection or comment. Dramatherapy is well positioned to assist here, with clear sessional definitions of beginning, middle and ending, including rituals that mark each phase and then the sending out of participants on the next journey. It is a mini-rehearsal for a life trajectory that ends at some point. John O'Donohue (2009) writes in *You are not going somewhere strange* about being unafraid, going home to the place we didn't leave, the going being protected and the spirit welcomed when it arrives. Thus life is a journey which ends and some have faith that it begins a new journey. Neil recognised this ending and continuum when the story character he role-played revealed to him he would not mind "return(ing) to the earth again" when he dies.

The inclusion of poetry in the book, to help with grief and dying, has been made on behalf of many people with dementia who are capable of reading still. An additional reason concerns the aesthetic opportunity it offers them of hearing and working with wise and rich language. Obviously, if the participant group is more diverse, it is essential to offer or encourage them to choose verse in their own languages. There are also questions too about a first language for immigrants, and how important it is for them to use the words they grew up with when the acquired language has all but disappeared from their memory.

Finally, the matter of assessment has been discussed in Chapter 10 along with commentary on scales and tools I used in the foundation project for this book. It is essential that our programs document our methods and techniques, and that our results are replicable, show considered outcomes and, most of all, are tailored to the developmental stages and situations of our participants.

It is significant to note that every professional has their own approach to their work, and it has been important to offer material that can be used by practitioners of dramatherapy and also other areas of allied health. The suggestions made in this book, creatively engaged with by the generous volunteers who agreed to take part in the research, can be adapted to other areas of therapy with elders and people with dementia.

References

Agli, O., Bailley, N., & Ferrand, C. (2014). Spirituality and religion in older adults with dementia: A systematic review. *International Psychogeriatrics*, *27*(5), 715–725.

Erikson, E. H. (1997). *The life cycle completed: Extended version by J. M. Erikson.* Norton & Co., Inc.

Gersie, A. (1991). *Storymaking in bereavement: Dragons fight in the meadow.* Jessica Kingsley.

Johnson, D. (2009). Developmental transformations: Towards the body as a presence. In D. Johnson & R. Emunah (Eds.), *Current approaches in dramatherapy* (pp. 89–116, 2nd ed.). Charles C. Thomas.

O'Donohue, J. (2009). *Anam cara: A book of Celtic wisdom*. Harper Collins.

Royal Commission into Aged Care Quality and Safety. (2019). Retrieved from https://agedcare.royalcommission.gov.au/publications/interim-report

Tornstam, L. (1997). Gerotranscendence: The contemplative dimension of aging. *Journal of Aging Studies, 11*(2), 143–154.

van der Kolk, B. (2015). *The body keeps the score: Mind, brain and body in the transformation of trauma*. Penguin Books.

Whyte, D. (2016, April 7). David Whyte: The conversational nature of reality [Podcast]. *On being*. Retrieved August 31, 2021 from https://onbeing.org/programs/david-whyte-the-conversational-nature-of-reality/

Afterword

It feels a real privilege to be invited to contribute the Afterword to this remarkable book. Joanna Jaaniste has thoroughly researched and written a very important work about dramatherapy with people with dementia, and it will be an essential text for many professional people, including therapists, who work in this field.

The book mainly focuses on an applied developmental model, Embodiment-Projection-Role (Jennings, 1999), applied with older people, and especially for those for whom it is necessary to improve their quality of life (QoL). Jaaniste has discovered that by reversing the sequence to Role-Projection-Embodiment (RPE), it is appropriate to the older stages of life and people's gradual disengagement with independent, lived experience.

There are some important early examples of developmental models of drama, including those conceived by Peter Slade (1954) and Richard Courtney (1981); both these distinguished people also pioneered methods of applied dramatherapy based on their drama connection with the life stages.

Slade (1954) maintained that drama conveys the personal growth and expression of each individual from childhood to adulthood. In child development, he distinguished two important play stages. In *Personal Play,* there is lots of movement, large and small, constant activity as a direct expression of the child. It is an expression incorporating the whole self. In *Projected Play,* there is an indirect imaginative energy transferred from the physical self into reading, drawing, painting, toy cars and dolls, for example. Whereas *Personal Play* is a spontaneous physical expression of the child's energy, *Projected Play* needs organisation and patience. One could consider both these early play stages as being reversed with the older people, with the energy and skills decreasing first and the personal play of movement expression being last to go.

Contrastingly, Richard Courtney (1981) has his own theory regarding drama and personality. He talks about the following:

1   "I am experience" – given through love, feeding, and handling; by the identification process.

2 "I do experience" – this is provided by play with what Courtney calls "mediate objects".

3 "I create experience" – This occurs with the primal act. This is the term that Courtney applies to the infant's first attempt at 10 months to impersonate and continues to grow and develop.

Courtney suggests that these stages recur throughout life and interestingly, he says, "Adults who doubt their abilities need to return to these steps – to engage in drama therapy" (p. 18).

Courtney also points out that drama is Social Action; that spontaneous drama is the way we relate to the world and improvisation in life creates our dynamic with others. I need no other to describe the essential qualities of Joanna Jaaniste's book than the thinking of these two great pioneers!

In the earlier part of the book, Jaaniste sets the context for her work and reminds us that very often, tests emphasise what older people cannot do rather than what they can do – the so called "disease model". There are assessments, such as Lahad's 6 Piece Story model (1992), which enable the dramatherapist to work in a skills model that encourages what a person can do, and it is important that the increased anxiety that people can experience in later life can be addressed through creative means. Jung, Erikson and others have emphasised the playfulness which can exist between the very young and the very old and draws our attention to the importance of spirituality for older people as a source of comfort, belief and support. Spiritual awareness does not necessarily mean religion, and individuals need to have choices about their spiritual practice.

Dramatherapists are able to provide not only life-enhancement methods but also end of life creative experience. Jaaniste describes how she uses poetry, both read as well as written, plus diaries, photos, letters, music and food in her work in "preparation of death" process. She describes how spectrograms and distancing can allow older people to bring their stories to life. Older people with dementia, as well as others, need to process their lived experiences, as well as their stories and anecdotes. The loss of close family members and friends needs to be acknowledged, and it may be that some people are "re-recognised" through photos. It is important that we can work with families and care staff to bring about an integrated approach. Often the dramatherapist can address issues that families may find too painful to deal with.

I want to end this Afterword with an example which endorses the approach in this book of believing the client in the moment and being able to work creatively with them. An 80-year woman with dementia would start shouting loudly late at night and banging on her bedroom door. The care staff would become very impatient and end up locking her door and ignoring her. A new carer, trained in drama, quietly went to her room and asked her why she was shouting, and she said, "I only want to go for a walk". He offered his arm in gallant style and she took his arm and off they went. They walked at a gentle pace down the corridor and into the next one. She then said, "I think that is far enough now, let's go home". So they turned and went back to her room, where she was tucked in and fell straight to sleep. No more shouting and no locked doors!

Throughout this text, we have ample case histories to illustrate theory and creative practice with older people, especially those with dementia. We have a detailed methodology for creative application and a host of ideas that are appropriate for older adults. The book gives us enthusiasm and a feeling of optimism that we can improve the QoL for people with dementia and use creative methods to maintain the creative parts of people's brains. They can receive respect and dignity and feel that they are accompanied appropriately at the end of their journey through life.

This is a remarkable book and one which I feel I can read, read again and discover treasures each time!

Dr Sue Jennings
Dramatherapy pioneer, Neuro-Dramatic-Play specialist
Professor of Play. Performer and Author.

References

Courtney, R. (1981). Drama assessment. In G. Schattner & R. Courtney (Eds.), *Drama in therapy* (Vol. 1, pp. 5–27). Drama Book Specialists.

Jennings, S. (1999). *Introduction to developmental playtherapy*. Jessica Kingsley.

Lahad, M. (1992). Story-making and assessment method for coping with stress: Six-piece story and BASICPh. In S. Jennings (Ed.), *Dramatherapy in theory and practice 2* (pp. 150–163). Tavistock Routledge.

Slade, P. (1954). *Child drama*. University of London Press.

Appendix

Session plan 1: Getting to know you

Objectives:
- Make a joint contract
- Participants demonstrate early cohesion by introductions and interaction
- Participants list their personal aims for the group
- Group members demonstrate understanding of warm-up activities
- Participants choose and reflect on photos, connecting with selves/group aims
- ' Participants assist in choice of ending ritual
  Contract and housekeeping
  Introductions in pairs

Warm-ups in the circle:

Name game – balls (Pass the ball and say the name of the recipient.)

Name game – gestures (Make a body gesture to the next one in the circle. The person mirrors it back, and then makes their own body gesture to the following member.)

Heads up: heads down (All participants listen to instruction – either "Heads down", which entails looking at the floor, or "Heads up", which means giving eye contact to another participant. If two people exchange eye contact, they exchange places.)

Choose a picture and discuss pictures in pairs (Photolanguage Australia, 1986).

Come into larger group and share aims, perceptions, memories.

Sing *Getting to know you* (Rodgers & Hammerstein, 1951).

Ending ritual – shake hands with the person next to you if you would like to.

Resources: iPod, balls, large photographs

Photolanguage Australia (1986). [Photographs]. Sydney Catholic Education Office.
Rodgers, R. (1951). (Composer). Hammerstein, O. (Writer). *Getting to know you.*
  Williamson Music.

Session plan 2: Seasons and weather

Objectives:
*   Remind about contract
*   Participants demonstrate early cohesion by further interaction
*   Participants list any other personal aims for the group
*   Group members demonstrate understanding of warm-up activities
*   Participants express in drawing, speech and movement how they feel
    about weather
*   Participants sing and assist in choice of ending ritual
    Reflection on last week's work
    Introductions (brief)

Warm-ups in the circle:

Name game – balls (similar to Session 1).
Ball pattern (Participants try to throw the ball to the same person each
    time and to receive the ball from the person who threw it to them.)
Clapping numbers (Participants clap together after each instruction –
    ONE (once); TWO (twice); THREE (three times) up until FIVE.
    Five is repeated, and then clapping resumes in a reverse direction
    back to ONE. One is repeated, and so on.)
Walking around in various weathers – Walk around the space and call
    out various types of weather. Pretend we are walking in that weather.
    Choose your favourite kind of weather. Sit with it for a moment,
    and then draw a picture of yourself in the weather. Facilitator will
    come around and tap you on the shoulder and then make a sound
    that goes with the weather, then a word or sentence.
Come into the middle if you can and make a shape of your body that
    connects with what you have just done – say what you see.
Find a partner and talk about your week. Then draw a line on another
    piece of paper – straight or wiggly or whatever your week was like.
    Draw weather for a part of your week.
Come into the group and reflect on your work and what you have
    drawn.
Listen to and sing *Just walking in the rain* (Johnston & Burke, 1936)
    and then sing *Getting to know you* (Rodgers & Hammerstein, 1951).
How would you like to end today?

Resources: iPod, balls, dry art materials

Johnston, A., & Burke, J. (Lyricists). (1936). E. Cohen (Producer) & N. Z. Mcleod (Director). *Pennies from heaven* [Motion Picture]. Columbia Pictures.

Rodgers, R. (1951). (Composer). Hammerstein, O. (Writer). *Getting to know you.* Williamson Music.

Session plan 3: Finding treasure

Objectives:
- Remind about contract
- Participants demonstrate early cohesion by further interaction
- Participants list varied names for feelings
- Group members demonstrate quicker uptake of warm-up activities
- Participants use objects as projective techniques to engage in storytelling
- Participants sing and assist in choice of ending ritual
  Reflection on last week's work

Warm-ups in circle:

> *Ball pattern* (as for previous session).
>
> *Clapping numbers* (as for previous session).
>
> *Shoo, fin, bounce* (*Shoo* is a gesture in a sweeping motion across the body, around the circle. Participants practise this one after another until they are accustomed to it. Then *fin* can be added, which sends the movement in the opposite direction. Participants can choose which named movement they send on. Once this gesture has been mastered, a third more complicated movement can be introduced known as *bounce*. The participant bounces on the spot, and the next participant gets missed, as the following one takes up the game. *Playback Theatre Game.* A. Lania (personal communication, September 9, 2010).)
>
> *How do you feel?* Walking around the room. Whenever a feeling is called out, make a shape with your body that corresponds with the feeling. Make a sound that goes with the feeling.
>
> *Group Mood.* Someone goes out of the room and the rest choose a mood.
>
> Try to act that mood and see if the person coming in from outside can guess what it is (Emunah, 1994, p. 148).
>
> Take an object from the lucky dip treasure box. Take your object and talk to a partner about it. Does it remind you of anything in particular?
>
> Share your object with the whole group and make a sculpt of it.
>
> Come into the group and talk or put into action what story it reminded you of.
>
> Everyone sings *Getting to know you* (Rodgers & Hammerstein, 1951).
>
> End with mirrored gestures.

Resources: iPod, various objects from 50s, 60s, balls, bag or basket to contain them

Emunah, R. (1994). *Acting for real.* Brunner Mazel Publishers.
Rodgers, R. (1951). (Composer). Hammerstein, O. (Writer). *Getting to know you.* Williamson Music.

Session plan 4: Colour

Objectives:
- Remind about contract
- Participants demonstrate early cohesion by further interaction
- Participants say how they are feeling
- Group members demonstrate attitudes to colour
- Participants choose a colour and stay with it to paint and perform
- Participants sing and assist in choice of ending ritual
  Reflection on how people feel
  Talk about colour – one sentence each

Warm-ups in the circle:

> *Ball pattern*
> *Clapping numbers*
> *Using cloths for improvisation* (A cloth is used by each person in turn – a participant can wear it or wave it in a certain way, use it as a beach towel, a picnic rug, or another option of their choice before passing it on. As with the gesture-passing in the previous session, each participant's creative contribution is mirrored after the cloth has been passed on. Once this has been done, a new innovation is made by that person, and so on around the circle.)
> Paint and show (one minute each).
> Perform, using paintings as inspiration for your performance.
> Reflect on performance.
> Everyone sings *Getting to know you* (Rodgers & Hammerstein, 1951).
> Ending – group choice.

Resources: iPod, paints, water, brushes, large sheets of paper, large balls, silk cloths

Rodgers, R. (1951). (Composer). Hammerstein, O. (Writer). *Getting to know you.* Williamson Music.

Session plan 5: Planting seeds

Objectives:
- Remind about contract
- Participants demonstrate embodiment and voice expression

- Participants say how they are feeling
- Group members tell us about their own experiences of planting seeds
- Participants mime their story
- Participants sing and assist in choice of ending ritual
  Reflection on how people feel.
  Talk growth – one sentence each.

Warm-ups:

Walking round room and leading with different parts of the body
Making shapes of various types of trees
Voicing sounds and feelings of those trees
Movement to music
Pick up cards – talk in pairs about planting seeds in your life.
Sculpt in pairs, respectfully turning your partner's body into a statue
   by suggesting change and asking permission to move an arm, etc.
   Take in turns to do so.
Join into fours and perform with sound and movement, using individ-
   ual body sculpts and harmonising them within your group.
Reflect on work, planting crocus bulbs in named pots and giving your
   bulb a message re future growth.
Everyone sings *Getting to know you* (Rodgers & Hammerstein,
   1951).
Ending – group choice.

Resources: iPod, silk cloths, crocus bulbs, named pots filled with soil, cards
with messages about planting seeds, e.g. "letting go", "growing tall", etc.

Rodgers, R. (1951). (Composer). Hammerstein, O. (Writer). *Getting to know you.*
   Williamson Music.

Session plan 6: The joys and woes of memory

Objectives:
- Remind about contract
- Participants demonstrate storytelling about their lives
- Participants say how they are feeling
- Group members walk through their life story remembering happenings
- Participants walk back through life stages, harvesting the gifts of those
  memories
- Participants freeze moments from the memories
- Participants sing "Thanks for the Memory"
  Reflection on how people feel.
  Memory – one sentence each.

Warm-ups in circle:

> *Shoo, fin, bounce* – Playback Theatre game. A. Lania (personal com-munication September 9, 2010)
>
> *Counting around circle*
>
> *Developmental Transformations* (Johnson et al., 2003)
>
> Go and visit each part of the room which represents an age – Childhood, Adolescence, 20–30, 30–50, 50–60+. Each area of the room is labelled as *Childhood, Young Adult, Marriage, Children, Grandchildren,* etc. Objects and pictures have been placed in each area. Each partici-pant has a small basket in which they can collect any object which appeals to them or reminds them of an incident in their life.
>
> Walk back through the stages, picking up pictures, cloths and objects. Reflect on these memories and freeze the actions.
>
> Everyone sings *Thanks for the Memory* (Robin & Rainger, 1938).
>
> Ending – group sends a "Whooosh" of energy to men who are sepa-rated from their families and not given access to their children.

Resources: iPod, reminiscence objects, cloths

Johnson, D., Smith, A., & James, M. (2003). Developmental transformations in group therapy with the elderly. In C. E. Schaefer (Ed.), *Play therapy with adults* (pp. 78–103). John Wiley & Sons.

Robin, L., & Rainger, R. (1938). Thanks for the memory. Retrieved June 6, 2012, from http://www.lyricsdepot.com/shep-fields/thanks-for-the-memory.html

Session plan 7: Grief and loss

Objectives:
- Remind about contract
- Participants demonstrate storytelling about their lives
- Participants say how they are feeling
- Group members remember losses and griefs
- Participants improvise/draw memories of these losses
- Participants freeze moments from the memories
- Participants sing "We'll meet again"
  Reflection on how people feel.
  Grief and loss memories – introduction to grief table.

Warm-ups:

> *Trust exercise* (Participants find a partner, and one is blindfolded while the other leads the "blind" partner around the room holding him firmly, while the therapist and others watch for possible obstacles.

Leaders are encouraged to check in with the "led", to see whether they are feeling safe, insecure, wish to stop, and so on. After a few minutes, the partners exchange reflections on the exercise and exchange roles (Emunah, 1994, p. 173; Jennings, 1986, p. 41).)

Ball throwing (Voicing memories of grief and loss with each throw.)

Story of *Ulu and the breadfruit tree* (Gersie & King, 1990).

Improvise the story, taking on roles, guided by narrator.

Reflect on story and what it reminds us of. Place a flower or feather on the grief table.

Everyone sings *We'll meet again* (Charles, 1943).

Ending: Each person makes a body sculpt of how they are feeling now, and the other participants mirror it back to them.

Resources: iPod, scarves for blindfolds, ball, cloths and simple costumes, feathers and flowers, grief table

Charles, H. (1943). *We'll meet again*. Recorded by Vera Lynne. London: Decca Records.

Emunah, R. (1994). *Acting for real*. Brunner Routledge.

Gersie, A., & King, N. (1990). *Storymaking in education and therapy*. Jessica Kingsley.

Jennings, S. (1986). *Creative drama in group work*. Speechmark Publishing Ltd.

Session plan 8: Celebrating ourselves

Objectives:
• Remind about contract
• Participants demonstrate storytelling about their lives
• Participants say how they are feeling
• Group members celebrate each other
• Participants improvise/draw memories of past group activities
• Participants freeze moments from the sessions
• Participants sing
   Reflection on how people feel.
   Introduction to celebrating ourselves.

Warm-ups in the circle:

Balloon game (The balloon is passed under the chin from one person to the next, around the circle. Similar to *Pass the Orange* (Jennings, 1986, p. 82).)

Cat and Mouse (Scher & Verrall, 1975, pp. 20–21).

Grandmother's Footsteps (A game in which one player turns round often and without warning with the aim of catching the other players. Players creep slowly and quietly up to touch him or her on the back or to take possession of an item placed next to the "Grandmother". The person arriving first or taking the item becomes the next Grandmother.)

Cat and Dog in pairs (Each participant takes a partner and decides who will be the cat and who will be the dog. They "speak" to one another in cat and dog language and then change roles after several minutes.)

Developmental Transformations (Johnson et al., 2003).

Free improvisation and roleplay using various hats and scarves.

Reflection on characters emerging from the dressups.

Everyone sings *You're too marvellous* (Whiting & Mercer, 1937) and *Every time we say goodbye* (Porter, 1981, p. 205).

Ending ritual where participants walk around and congratulate one another on a special quality they possess.

Resources: iPod, balloons, variety of hats, cloths and scarves

Jennings, S. (1986). *Creative drama in group work*. Speechmark Publishing Ltd.

Johnson, D., Smith, A., & James, M. (2003). Developmental transformations in group therapy with the elderly. In C. E. Schaefer (Ed.), *Play therapy with adults* (pp. 78–103). John Wiley & Sons.

Porter, C. (1981). *Great American songbook*. Chappell & Co.

Scher, A., & Verrall, C. (1975). *100+ ideas for drama*. Heinemann Educational Publishers.

Whiting, R., & Mercer, J. (1937). *You're too marvellous*. G. & C. Merriam, Co.

Session plan 9: Animal kingdom

Objectives:
*   Remind about contract
*   Participants demonstrate storytelling about their lives
*   Participants say how they are feeling
*   Group members show improvisational skills
*   Participants use games, impro and pictures as stimulus material for clay modelling
*   Participants sing *Tie me kangaroo down, sport* (Harris, 1960)
    Reflection on how people feel.
    Introduction to animals in our lives.

Warm-ups in the circle:

Ball game (This could be a ball pattern or a name game, depending on how the group is feeling after a three-week break.)

Mirroring clapping game (Building on the earlier 1–5 clapping game, individuals clap a rhythm which is then mirrored by others in the circle.)

Cat and Mouse (Scher & Verrall, 1975)

Guess the animal (Cards bearing the names of animals are picked from a bag. There are two cards with the names of each animal. Each participant improvises their animal and finds their monkey or cat partner from their improvisation.)

Find your partner from impros.

Take some clay and model an animal, looking at pictures of animals if you wish.

Reflection.

Everyone sing *Tie me Kangaroo Down, Sport* (Harris, 1960).

Ending: Each participant mime an animal in the centre of the circle, and the other members mirror that mime back to them.

Resources: iPod, balls, cards, clay, water, sponges and cleaning cloths, boards for working clay

Harris, R. (1960). *Tie me kangaroo down sport.* [Audio Recording]. Epic. EMI Columbia.

Scher, A., & Verrall, C. (1975). *100+ ideas for drama.* Heinemann Educational Publishers.

Session plan 10: Magic shop

Objectives:
- Remembering last week
- Participants demonstrate spontaneity
- Participants express what they are looking for in life
- Group members disclose what they are willing to give up in exchange
- Participants sing "We'll meet again" (Charles, 1943)
  Reflection on how people feel and remembering last week.

Warm-ups in circle:

Guess what I'm doing (Standing in the circle, participants take turns to improvise an activity in the centre. The person who guesses the nature of the activity then takes the place of the first improviser.)

Diamonds (Participants form groups of four, choosing a leader. They stand in a diamond formation, all looking in the same direction with the leader at the apex. The leader makes active movements with limbs and body, and others copy them. The leader chooses the next leader to his right or left, and the other three turn to face the leader's back. The same routine applies until each member of the diamond has had a turn at leadership.)

Emotional machines (Drama games for kids, 2013).

Incidents improvised (A participant chooses others to improvise a memory on a theme with them: for example, "At the beach". The scene takes place, participants de-role and the instigator reflects briefly on the improvisation.)

Developmental Transformations (Johnson et al., 2003).

Take turns in the *Magic Shop*. More detail is given by Reneé Emunah (1994, pp. 220–222).

Reflection.

Everyone sings *We'll meet again* (Charles, 1943).

Ending: Take it in turns to wave a magic wand and give an instruction for the others – for example, everyone wave goodbye.

Resources: iPod, dressups, cloths

Charles, H. (1943). *We'll meet again*. Recorded by Vera Lynne. Decca Records.

Drama games for kids. (2013). Beat by Beat Press. Retrieved September 28, 2021, from https://www.bbbpress.com/2013/04/the-machine/

Emunah, R. (1994). *Acting for real*. Brunner Mazel Publishers.

Johnson, D., Smith, A., & James, M. (2003). Developmental transformations in group therapy with the elderly. In C. E. Schaefer (Ed.), *Play therapy with adults* (pp. 78–103). John Wiley & Sons.

Session plan 11: Dealing with difficult people

Objectives:
- Remembering last week
- Participants demonstrate openness about difficult people
- Participants improvise difficult people in their lives
- Group members reverse roles with the difficult person, if they can.
- Participants sing together
  Reflection on how people feel and remembering last week – cards with feelings.

Warm-ups in the circle:

Shoo, fin, bounce

Diamonds

Hand Game (This game is best played with participants seated on the floor or around a circular table. See *The Hand Game* (Ultimate Camp Resource, 2021).)

Sculptor and Statue (Similar to *Partner Sculpting* (Emunah, 1994, p. 157).)

Volunteers role-reversal. Participants take "difficult" roles in pairs.

Reflection.

Everyone sing *Near friends, dear friends* (Watts, 2006). (A different song had been planned for this session; however, it was inappropriate and cohesion was needed after difficult role-reversal and improvisations.)

Ending: Participants pass a mimed action to the next person in the circle. This is then changed into a new mimed action by the next person and passed on around the group.

Resources: iPod, circular table, dressups, cloths

Emunah, R. (1994). *Acting for real.* Brunner Mazel Publishers.

Ultimate camp resource (2021). [Video file]. Retrieved September 29, 2021, from https://www.ultimatecampresource.com/camp-videos/the-hand-game/

Watts, J. (2006). *A few songs occasioned by the Spirit.* Retrieved September 29, 2021, from http://jonwattsmusic.com/album/a-few-songs-occasioned

Session plan 12: In the land of forgetfulness

Objectives:
- Remembering last week
- Participants demonstrate awareness about memory being difficult for all
- Participants demonstrate spontaneity in the play space
- Group members show they can transform fear, anger, tears and emptiness
- Participants sing *Near friends, dear friends* (Watts, 2006)
- Leanne to play a tune on piano, if she can (prepare before group)
  Reflection on how people feel and remembering last week – cards with feelings.

Warm-ups in the circle:

Fruit Bowl (Put chairs in a circle. Turn one chair to face out. Name each participant apple, pear, banana around circle. There will be at least two of each fruit. Choose someone to stand in the middle. They (or you) can call apple (or) pear (or) banana. If the name applies to a participant, they must get up and change places. The caller finds a seat. The last participant is left standing, becomes the new caller. No one can change places with the person sitting next to them. If "Fruit Bowl" is called, everyone changes places.)

Adam and Eve (Scher & Verrall, 1975, p. 24).

Touch Game (Scher & Verrall, 1975, p. 55).

Developmental Transformations: the Land of Forgetfulness – finding anger, fear, emptiness & tears (Macy & Brown, 1998, p. 101).

Bringing back gifts from the Land – Reflection on transformation of objects.

Everyone sing *Near friends, dear friends* (Watts, 2006).

Ending: Participants send a hand-squeeze around the group.

Resources: stones, sticks, leaves and bowls; silk cloths

Macy, J., & Brown, Y. (1998). *Coming back to life: Practices to reconnect our lives, our world.* New Society Publishers.

Scher, A., & Verrall, C. (1975). *100+ ideas of drama.* Heinemann Educational Publishers.

Watts, J. (2006). *A few songs occasioned by the Spirit.* Retrieved September 29, 2021, from http://jonwattsmusic.com/album/a-few-songs-occasioned

Session plan 13: Joys and woes of memory

Objectives:
* Remembering last week
* Participants demonstrate awareness about memory being difficult for all
* Participants demonstrate awareness of olfactory memory
* Group members show they can create vignettes from memories of scent
* Participants sing *Thanks for the memory* (Robin & Rainger, 1938)
* Leanne to play a tune on piano, if she can (prepare before group) Reflection on how people feel and remembering last week.

Warm-ups in the circle:

Stretchy cloth dance to music.

Who started the motion? (Emunah, 1994, p. 181).

Emotion machine (Drama games for kids, 2021). (A participant starts the motion of an "emotion machine". Each further participant, in turn, takes a role in making the machine function. The emotion can be decided beforehand, or each participant can use their own initiative to support the emotional build-up.)

I remember when … (A player finishes this sentence and the others have to quickly form the scene the person remembers – group sculpt which can morph into improv.)

Smelling Game. Choose a partner, and each person has a pen and chart. Pick up the numbered smelling bags off the cloth, one by one, and fill in the spaces below the numbers on the chart once you have smelled the bag.

Bring back to group, and share the memories the scents brought up – more freeze scenes.

Reflect on work.

Choose three favourite smells, whether or not they are part of the game.
Sing: *Thanks for the memory* (Robin & Rainger, 1938).
Sing: *Near friends, dear friends* (Watts, 2006).
Ending: Participants send a hand-squeeze around the group.

Resources: smelling bags, blindfolds, large stretchy cloth, silk cloths, templates to complete, pens

Emunah, R. (1994). *Acting for real.* Brunner Mazel.
Drama games for kids. (2013). Beat by Beat Press. Retrieved September 28, 2021, from https://www.bbbpress.com/2013/04/the-machine/
Robin, L., & Rainger, R. (1938). *Thanks for the memory.* Retrieved September 28, 2001, from http://www.lyricsdepot.com/shep-fields/thanks-for-the-memory.html
Watts, J. (2006). *A few songs occasioned by the Spirit.* Retrieved September 28, 2021, from http://jonwattsmusic.com/album/a-few-songs-occasioned

Session plan 14: Past, present and future

Objectives:
* Remembering last week
* Participants collaborate with others' memories
* Participants think about what they would like for the future
* Participants sing *"Thanks for the memory"*
* L to play a tune on piano, if she can (prepare before group)
  Reflection on how people feel and remembering last week.

Warm-ups in the circle:

> *Fruit Bowl* (See Session 12.)
> *Finding your strength in partners.* (Partners place the flat of their two hands against their partners'. They press against one another, using their body weight, but without trying to knock each other over! The idea is to test their strength together.)
> *Tug of war.*
> *Cat and mouse* (Scher & Verrall, 1975, p. 20).

Scenarios from last week:

> N being in the kitchen while his mother is cooking as a child.
> L's memory of Christmas.
> D's memory of the orchard and being in trouble.
> What do people want for the future? Throw ball with wishes for future. Dramatherapist writes them on cards. Walk around to see them on cards. Draw your wish for the future and share.

Sing: *Thanks for the memory* (Robin & Rainger, 1938).

Sing: *Near friends, dear friends* (Watts, 2006).

Ending: Participants take an object from an imaginary box in the centre of the circle, and give it to another member of the group, telling them what it is. Participants are advised to give something appropriate for that person, from what they know of them.

Resources: cloths, art materials

Robin, L., & Rainger, R. (1938). *Thanks for the memory.* Retrieved September 28, 2001, from http://www.lyricsdepot.com/shep-fields/thanks-for-the-memory.html

Scher, A., & Verrall, C. (1975). *100+ ideas for drama.* Heinemann Educational Publishers.

Watts, J. (2006). *A few songs occasioned by the Spirit.* Retrieved September 28, 2021, from http://jonwattsmusic.com/album/a-few-songs-occasioned

Session plan 15: Grief and loss

Objectives:
*   Remembering last week
*   Participants say how they are feeling
*   Group members remember losses and griefs
*   Participants improvise memories of these losses
*   Participants sing "We'll meet again"
    Reflection on how people feel.
    Grief and loss memories – losses.

Warm-ups:

Trust walk (Emunah, 1994, p. 173).

Stuck in the Mud (Jennings, 1986, p. 86).

Tag Game (Active for Life, 2021).

Pick up a twig and do a brief drawing of the tree that it came from – place near grief table.

Write on a card something about a promise that has been made – perhaps broken – or a loss that has occurred in your life and place the card near a drawing that you like.

Talk about a loss that you have experienced or a promise that has been broken.

Opportunity for dramatherapy work with someone's loss.

Sing *We'll meet again* (Charles, 1943).

Sing *Near friends, dear friends* (Watts, 2006).

Ending: Each participant goes into the centre of the circle and body sculpts a gesture, whereupon the other members mirror it back to them.

Resources: twigs from a tree, dry art materials, plain cards, A3 paper

Active for Life (2021). *Ten fun ways you can transform the game of tag.* Retrieved September 30, 2021, from https://activeforlife.com

Charles, H. (1943). *We'll meet again.* Recorded by Vera Lynne. Decca Records.

Emunah, R. (1994). *Acting for real.* Brunner Mazel.

Jennings, S. (1986). *Creative drama in group work.* Speechmark Publishing Ltd.

Watts, J. (2006). *A few songs occasioned by the Spirit.* Retrieved September 28, 2021, from http://jonwattsmusic.com/album/a-few-songs-occasioned

Session plan 16: Bringing gifts to the feast

Objectives:
- Clients express appreciation for one another.
- Clients choose an activity, gesture or a few words in order to remember what we have done together.
- Clients are empowered to engage with different types of memory: semantic, episodic, emotional and procedural.
  Reflection on how people feel and last week.
  Talk about Bringing Gifts to the Feast.

Warm-ups:

> *Magic Box* (Go into the playspace for the last time, where there is a magic box. Find a quality or a feeling in there, and keep it, or give it to someone. Then re-enact anything you remember from what we have done in the 16 sessions. Then step out of playspace.)
>
> Take a fruit or a flower, and put it in a bowl in the centre. Does it symbolise something for you?
>
> Sing *We'll meet again* (Charles, 1943).
>
> Sing *Near friends, dear friends* (Watts, 2006).
>
> Ending: make a sound or say a word and a body sculpt, which can say goodbye to the group and can be mirrored by them.

Resources: fruit and flowers

Return plants participants bedded in pots at morning tea.

Charles, H. (1943). *We'll meet again.* Recorded by Vera Lynne. Decca Records.

Watts, J. (2006). *A few songs occasioned by the Spirit.* Retrieved September 28, 2021, from http://jonwattsmusic.com/album/a-few-songs-occasioned

Index